Liljana Bogdanovska
Rumenka Petkovska

Evaluation of betamethasone dipropionate therapeutic level in GCF

Liljana Bogdanovska
Rumenka Petkovska

Evaluation of betamethasone dipropionate therapeutic level in GCF

Development of RP-HPLC method for determination of betamethasone dipropionate in gingival crevicular fluid

LAP LAMBERT Academic Publishing

Imprint

Any brand names and product names mentioned in this book are subject to trademark, brand or patent protection and are trademarks or registered trademarks of their respective holders. The use of brand names, product names, common names, trade names, product descriptions etc. even without a particular marking in this work is in no way to be construed to mean that such names may be regarded as unrestricted in respect of trademark and brand protection legislation and could thus be used by anyone.

Cover image: www.ingimage.com

Publisher:
LAP LAMBERT Academic Publishing
is a trademark of
International Book Market Service Ltd., member of OmniScriptum Publishing Group
17 Meldrum Street, Beau Bassin 71504, Mauritius

ISBN: 978-3-659-20397-8

Copyright © Liljana Bogdanovska, Rumenka Petkovska
Copyright © 2014 International Book Market Service Ltd., member of OmniScriptum Publishing Group

TABLE OF CONTENTS

1. INTRODUCTION 3
2. PERIODONTAL DISEASE: BACKGROUND 4
2.1 Immuno-inflammatory processes in perodontal disease 7
3. GINGIVAL CREVICULAR FLUID 9
4. GCF COLLECTION METHODS 12
4.1 Gingival washing techniques 12
4.2 Collection of GCF by using capillary tubes or micropipettes 13
4.3 Collection of GCF by using absorbent paper strips 13
5. THERAPEUTIC APPROACHES IN PERIODONTAL DISEASE 17
5.1 Corticosteroids as therapeutic modality in periodontal disease 19
5.2. Betamethasone dipropionate as adjunct to periodontal treatment 24
5.3 Methods for the analysis of corticosteroid molecules in biological samples 25
5.4 RP-HPLC methods in periodontal therapeutic drug monitoring 28
6. AIM OF THE STUDY 30
7. MATERIALS AND METHODS 32
7.1 Materials 32
7.2 Gingival crevicular fluid (GCF) samples 32
7.3 Human serum samples 32
7.4 Chemical and reagents 32
7.5 Instrumentation 32
7.6 Chromatographic conditions 33
7.7 Collection of GCF samples 33

7.8	Preparation of standard solutions and quality control (QC) samples 34
7.9	GCF sample preparation 34
7.10	Bioanalytical method validation 36
8.	RESULTS AND DISCUSSION 39
8.1	Optimization of a RP-HPLC method for determination of BDP in GCF 41
8.1.1	Considerations for the method development 41
8.1.2	Identification of BDP and IS in GCF sample 43
8.1.3	Optimization of the mobile phase composition and flow rate 43
8.1.4	Selection of suitable wavelength of detection 44
8.1.5	Optimization of the buffer concentration 44
8.1.6	Optimization of the injection volume 45
8.1.7	Selection of the column temperature 45
8.1.8	Selection of the internal standard 45
8.1.9	Optimization of the sample pretreatment procedure for determination of BDP in GCF samples 47
8.2	Bioanalytical method validation 49
8.2.1	Selectivity 49
8.2.2	Linearity 51
8.2.3	Accuracy and precision 52
8.2.4	Recovery 54
8.2.5	Stability 55
8.2.6	Analysis of patient GCF samples 56
9.	CONCLUSION 63
10.	REFERENCE 67

1. INTRODUCTION

Periodontal disease is a general term that encompasses several pathological conditions affecting the protective and supportive structures of the teeth (Schwach-Abdellaou et al., 2000; Shaddox & Walker, 2010). These conditions are characterized by destruction of the periodontal ligament, resorption of the alveolar bone and apical migration of the junctional epithelium along the tooth surface, which results in periodontal pocket formation (Schwach-Abdellaou et al., 2000; Zia et al., 2011).

Data obtained from various epidemiological studies indicate that periodontal disease affects virtually all adult individuals resulting in decreased quality of life and increased health-care cost. Approximately 70% of the US adult population is affected by any kind of periodontitis with prevalence rates and severity higher among men than women and among blacks than whites (Horz & Conrads, 2007). Recent work has shown that several systemic diseases might also be linked to the presence of periodontitis (Kantarci & Van Dyke, 2005). As periodontal disease tends to disturb the integrity of oral mucous membranes, periodontal pathogens can enter the systemic circulation and become serious and significant challenge to the entire human body. These bacterial "attacks", together with the host's inflammatory reaction, may not only cause bacteriemia but also (under certain circumstances) septicemia, organ apcesses or endocarditis, as well as other cardiovascular disorders and low birth weight when occurring during pregnancy. Furthermore, if left untreated, periodontitis increases the risk for serious cardiovascular diseases and cerebrovascular diseases and stroke (Horz & Conrads, 2007).

Having in mind serious adverse effects that periodontal disease can have on human health, effective periodontal therapy is needed. The aim of the current periodontal therapy is to retain periodontal health by decreasing inflammation and by reducing the periodontal pocket depth. This is mostly achieved by mechanical procedures, scaling and root planning (SRP), and surgery in some cases (Schwach-Abdellaou et al., 2000). However, in most cases, locally or systemically antimicrobials or corticosteroids must be applied as adjuncts to scaling and root planning.

Locally applied corticosteroids are used routinely in clinical praxis as adjunct to scaling and root planning. They act as the host's modulatory agents and represent a therapeutical modality in the current periodontal therapy (Fachin & Zaki, 1991; Seymor, 2006; Aras et al., 2007).

Current literature data suggest that several drugs are excreted and concentrated in the gingival crevicular fluid (GCF), inflammatory exudates closely related to periodontal disease activity. These drugs can be advantageously used in the periodontal treatment. Developing new, sensitive and selective methods for their determination and quantification in GCF and other oral fluids will be of special interest to the dental practitioners and will enable close monitoring and evaluation of the periodontal treatment.

2. PERIODONTAL DISEASE: BACKGROUND

Chronic infectious diseases of the oral cavity in human population can be divided in two general categories: dental caries and periodontal disease. Dental caries is a progressive irreversible microbial disease affecting the hard parts of the tooth. Once it occurs, the lesions persist throughout life even if the lesion is treated (Kinney et al., 2007).

Periodontal diseases are the most important chronic infections that lead to chronic inflammation, which results in host-mediated destruction of the supporting tissues of the dentition (Kornman et al., 1997). Periodontal diseases can be divided into reversible and nonreversible categories. Gingivitis is a reversible inflammatory reaction of the marginal gingiva to dental plaque biofilms. It is characterized by an intial increase in the blood flow, enhanced vascular permeability and influx of polymorphonuclear leukocytes [PMNs] and macrophages from the peripheral blood into the periodontal connective tissue. Changes in the soft tissues of the periodontium in gingivitis include redness, edema, bleeding and tenderness. The feature distinguishing gingivitis from the destructive form of periodontal disease is the intact anatomical location of the junctional epithelium. Epidemiological studies indicate that gingivitis of varying severity is nearly universal in children and adolescents. These studies also indicate that the prevalence of destructive forms of periodontal disease is lower in younger individuals than in adults. Despite the low prevalence of periodontitis in children and adolescents, they should receive periodic periodontal evaluation as a component of routine dental visits (Kinney et al., 2007).

Periodontitis, i.e., "peri" = around, "odont"= tooth, "itis" = inflammation, the destructive category of periodontal disease, is a nonreversible inflammatory state of the supporting structures of the teeth (Kantarci & Van Dyke, 2005). It is one of the most widespread diseases of mankind. After its initiation, the disease progresses with the loss of collagen fibers, and attachment to the cemental surface, apical migration of the pocket epithelium, formation of deepened periodontal pockets, and resorption of alveolar bone (Fig. 1). If left untreated, the disease continues to progressive bone destruction, leading to tooth mobility and subsequent tooth loss (Kinney et al., 2007). Chronic periodontitis is most prevalent in adults. It can be localized (less than 30% of the dentition affected) or generalized (more than 30 % of the dentition affected). Furthermore, the severity of the disease can be mild (1 to 2 mm clinical attachment loss), moderate (3 to 4 mm clinical attachment loss), or severe (more than 5 mm clinical attachment loss). According to epidemiological data, the occurrence of periodontal diseases is related to the oral hygiene status and the socio-economic class

(Alvarez et al., 2011). In the United States, the prevalence of chronic periodontitis in adults is around 35% (Albandar, 2002), whereas in Western Europe 13-54% of the population is affected by periodontal diseases (Sheiham, 2005). In low-income countries, the percentage of the population affected is around 45% (Hamasha et al., 2000; Attin et al., 1999; Page et al., 1997).

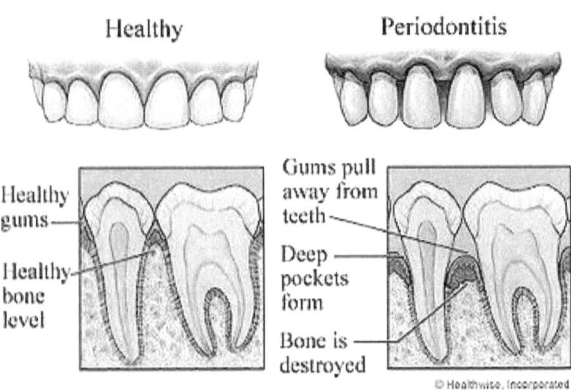

Figure 1. Tissues of the periodontium in health and in periodontitis

The individual's susceptibility to periodontitis can be affected by a number of environmental and acquired risk factors like heredity, smoking, hormonal variation (during pregnancy, menopause), systemic diseases (Marfan's and Ehler-Danlos syndromes, diabetes, osteoporosis, HIV, neutropenias), stress, nutritional deficiencies, medications (calcium channel blockers, immunomodulatory agents or anticonvulsants) and poor oral hygiene (Tariq et al., 2012).

Within the sophisticated system of tissues of the periodontium, the teeth serve not only as a medium for external stimuli, but its surface is also an environment for the accumulation and colonization by a diverse group of bacterial species (Kantarci and Van Dyke, 2005). More than 600 different bacteria are capable of colonizing the human mouth. It has been estimated that approximately 10% play a causal role in the initiation of periodontal disease. Three organisms in particular have been directly associated with chronic periodontits, *Tanerella forsythensis, Porphyromonas gingivalis and Treponema denticola* (Kinney et al., 2007).

Once bacteria are attached to the hard and soft surfaces of the teeth, the host responds with various forms of defense machinery (Offenbacher, 1996). The interaction between the dental-periodontal tissues and invading organisms is a life-long process that begins immediately after tooth eruption. Thus, periodontitis can be described as an impaired balance between the host's defense mechanisms and colonizing microorganisms (Kantarci & Van Dyke, 2005).

2.1 Immuno-inflammatory processes in perodontal disease

Periodontal disease is a complex chronic inflammatory disease of the oral cavity. It is typical for all complex diseases that vary in the age of one-set and are linked to multiple biological pathways and multiple genetic and environmental factors (Loos and Thoja, 2005).

Our understanding of the etiology of periodontal disease has progressed by leaps and bounds over the past 50 years. Early theories focused on the fact that the bacteria were the only responsible factor for the occurrence of the periodontal disease. They were believed to release enzymes and toxins that destroyed the periodontium. This is referred to as the non-specific plaque hypothesis. A specific plaque hypothesis, the understanding that specific types of bacteria, not just the plaque accumulation, caused the disease developed from this view. Today, the bacterial plaque is referred to as bacterial biofilm and the periodontal disease is defined as a biofilm-associated inflammatory disease by multiple ethiologies (Berezov & Darveau, 2011).

The pathogenesis of periodontal disease is characterized by local and systemic inflammatory response to the microbial biofilm. The microbial challenge stimulates the host response, which results in disease limited to the gingival (gingivitis) or initiation of periodontitis. Perpetuation of the host response due to persistent bacterial challenge disrupts the homeostatic mechanisms and results in recruitment of neutrophils, macrophages and release of mediators such as pro-inflammatory cytokines, matrix metalloproteinases, arachidonic acid metabolites, reactive oxygen species as well as release of mediators for osteoclastic bone resorption. Protective aspects of the host's response include recruitment of neutrophils, production of protective antibodies, and possibly release of anti-inflammatory cytokines including the transforming factor-β, interleukin-4 (IL-4), IL-10 and IL-11 (Kornman et al., 1997).

Cytokines are inflammatory mediators that stimulate fibroblasts and epithelial cells to release prostaglandins (PGE_2) and matrix metalloproteinase. Constituents of the biofilm stimulate the host cells to produce pro-inflammatory cytokines including interleukin-1β, IL-6 and tumor necrosis factor-α (TNF-α), which may induce connective tissue and alveolar bone destruction. The prostaglandins induce alveolar bone loss while matrix metalloproteinases, also known as collagenases, damage or destroy the connective tissue (Kirkwood et al., 2007).

This thorough understanding of the host's inflammatory response in periodontal pathogenesis presents an opportunity for new treatment strategies by means of host response modulation (Kirkwood et al., 2007; Souza et al., 2010).

3. GINGIVAL CREVICULAR FLUID

Periodontal pockets are one of the most important clinical signs of periodontal disease activity. They can be defined as deepening of the gingival sulcus as a result of apical migration of the junctional epithelium due to inflammatory changes in the connective tissue wall of the gingival sulcus. Pockets also contain food reminants, salivary mucin, desquamed epithelial cells, leucocytes and gingival crevicular fluid (Patel, 2010). Of the three fluids that can be found in the oral cavity – serum, total saliva and gingival crevicular fluid (GCF), the last one has been the center of attention in recent years (Koss et al., 2009).

Gingival crevicular fluid is an osmotically mediated inflammatory exudate or altered serum transudate originating from the gingival plexus of blood vessels in the gingival corium, subjacent to the epithelium lining of the dentogingival space (Kavadia-Tsatala et al., 2002). The formation of GCF is presented in Fig. 2. Its presence has attracted the attention of many researchers since the 19th century. Waerhaug (1952), Brill and Krasse (1958) are the earliest pioneer workers who analyzed the volume, composition and role of GCF in defense mechanism of the oral cavity (Patel, 2010).

The biochemical composition of GCF (Fig. 3) resembles that of serum and the intensity of its flow has been shown to vary as a function of gingival inflammation (Koss et al., 2009). It can be said, that GCF composition is a result of a complex interplay between bacterial biofilm adherent to tooth surfaces and the cells of the periodontal tissues (Champagne at al., 2003).

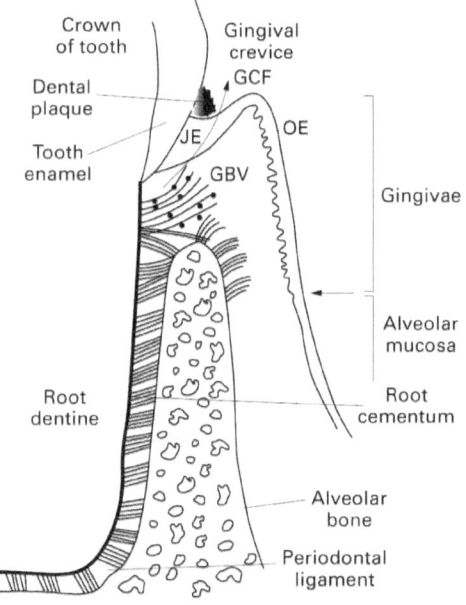

Figure 2. Schematic diagram of periodontal tissues and GCF formation

GCF contains electrolytes in concentrations similar to plasma (potassium, calcium), cellular elements (desquamated epithelial cells, bacteria and leukocytes), organic compounds (glucose hexamine, hexuronic acid), metabolic and bacterial products (lactic acid, urea, prostaglandins and hydrogen sulfide) as well as enzyme and enzyme inhibitors (alkaline phosphatase, β-glucoronudase, hyaluronidase, collagenases and lactic acid serum proteinase inhibitors). The total protein content of the GCF is much less than that of serum. GCF contains albumin, globulins, protease inhibitors, and components of the complement. GCF has a protective role in the defense mechanism of the oral cavity by removing potential harmful products, molecules and pathogens, and also has an antibacterial role containing pathogen neutralizing antibodies (Malamud & Rodrigues-Chaves, 2011).

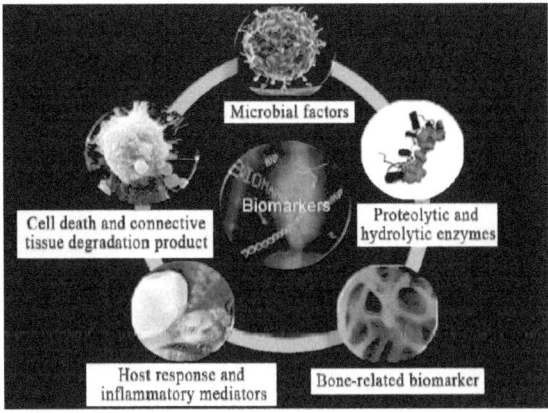

Figure 3. Biochemical composition of gingival crevicular fluid

As an exudate, GCF reflects metabolic changes in periodontal tissues. As it traverses through inflamed periodontal tissues, it is believed to pick up enzymes and other molecules that participate in the destructive processes as well as products of cell and tissue degradation (Malhotra et al., 2010).

Since crevicular fluid seems to be a characteristic feature of gingival and periodontal inflammation, one can reasonably expect that when suitable therapeutic agents are given to the patient, they can be carried from the systemic circulation to the gingival sulcus/periodontal pocket by flow of the fluid (Reddy, 2008). It has been shown that several drugs such as chlorhexidine (Soskolne et al., 1998), tinidazole (Liew et al., 1991), metronidazole (Pahkla et al., 2005), tetracycline (Vinneau & Kindberg, 1997) and ciprofloxacin (Dincel et al., 2005) achieve therapeutic concentrations and can be measured in GCF.

In conclusion, it can be said that the origin, the composition and the clinical significance of GCF are now well known and documented. All of these data have significantly helped in understanding the periodontal disease etiology and progression. It is now obvious that chemical and biochemical analysis of GCF provides unique possibilities in monitoring different periodontal conditions.

4. GCF COLLECTION METHODS

The presence and the volume of GCF can be indicative of changes to periodontal tissues that are a consequence of the inflammatory response of the host, triggered by aggression from the dental biofilm (Linden et al., 2002). As inflammatory exudate, GCF contains biological markers, inflammatory mediators and antibodies that originate from connective tissues (Loos & Thoja, 2005). GCF is constantly secreted, initiating before structural periodontal changes can be detected by physical means (Del Fabro et al., 2001).

The collection of GCF can be a relatively easy and non invasive procedure. This is of special importance regarding the fact that the analysis of the specific components in GCF provides a quantitative biochemical indicator for the evaluation of the local cellular metabolism that reflects a person's periodontal health status.

GCF can be collected by a variety of methods such as suction (using capillary tubes or micropipettes), lavage (gingival washing technique) or absorption paper strips (Griffiths at al., 2003). The technique chosen will primarily depend upon study objectives.

4.1 Gingival washing techniques

Gingival washing techniques have been employed for harvesting different types of cells from the gingival crevice region. In this technique, the periodontal pocket is perfused with an isotonic solution such as Hank's balanced solution, usually of a fixed volume. The fluid collected then represents a dilution of GCF and contains both cells and soluble constituents such as plasma proteins (Patel, 2010). Unfortunately, this method for collecting the GCF suffers from several disadvantages. First of all, it is technically demanding which limits its use to only few individuals. The GCF from individual sites cannot be analyzed, but the major disadvantage is the fact that all the fluid may not be recovered during the aspiration and re-aspiration procedure. Thus, the accurate quantification of GCF volume or composition is not possible as the precise volume cannot be determined.

4.2 Collection of GCF by using capillary tubes or micropipettes

For collection of predetermined volumes of GCF, microcappilary tubules or micropipettes are placed at the gingival crevice and either held at a particular site or passed forth and back for 10-15 minute periods. This procedure can often be disruptive to the delicate crevicular epithelium, resulting in contamination of the native GCF with blood and serum. Collection of significant, predetermined volumes can also cause an influx of serum from gingival capillaries, leading to a dilution of the native GCF by serum, since the usual volume range in the undisturbed sulcus is between 0.5 and 1µL (Vinneay & Kindberg, 1997; Kavadia-Tsatala et al., 2002).

4.3 Collection of GCF by using absorbent paper strips

The method for collecting GCF using absorbent paper strips is one the most commonly used methods in GCF analysis. The paper strips are placed in the gingival crevice (Kavadia-Tsatala et al., 2002) and in this way, GCF migrates from the crevice to the paper strip via capillary action. It is easy to carry out, requires minimal operating skills and compared to the methods mentioned above, it is practically non-invasive (Griffiths, 2003). Although each method for GCF collection has its own advantages and disadvantages, collection with absorbent paper strips is one of the most frequent methods found in literature.

Several different types of absorbent paper strips are commercially available and have been assessed previously: Durapore, Millipore (Giannopolou et al., 2003), Whatman chromatographic paper 2x5mm or 2x6mm (Johnson et al., 1999) and absorbent paper strips (Serra et al., 2003). However, the reference absorbent paper widely recognized as the method of choice for GCF collection via absorption is the Periopaper® (Deinzer et al., 2000; Ozkavaf et al., 2001).

In the most commonly employed method, the sample area is isolated in order to minimize the possibility of saliva contamination and gently dried with air. Then the absorbable paper strip can be placed into or laid outside the gingival crevice. The extracrevicular technique involves overlaying the strip on the gingival crevice region in an attempt to minimize trauma (Fig. 4b). In contrast, using the intracrevicular method, the paper strip is inserted into the entrance of the gingival crevice until minimal resistance is felt (Fig. 4a).

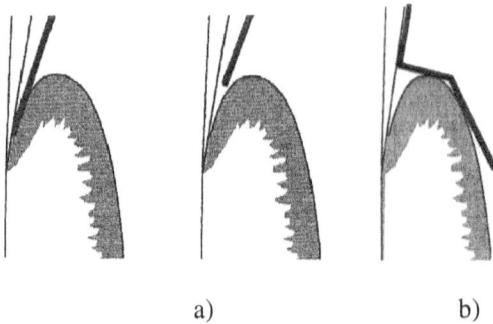

a)   b)

Figure 4. Intracrevicular (a) and extracrevicular (b) techniques for GCF collection

The collection time can vary between 30-60 seconds. The collection time of 30 seconds is used most commonly because in this manner the probability for blood contamination is decreased. However, the optimal GCF collection time must be carefully chosen because short duration for sample collection may result in GCF volumes that cannot be quantified with Periotron 6000®. According to Figuero & Gustaffson (1998), one of the major advantages of using absorption to collect GCF is the possibility to measure its volume, which leads to the discussion of the best way of reporting the components of this exudate. It has been suggested that GCF components can be reported as total quantities (mg), concentrations (ng mL^{-1}) and collection time (Ciantar & Caruana, 1998; Griffiths, 2003; Hanioka et al., 2005).

Although some authors claim that the fluid volume is dependent on inflammation present at the diseased site (Del Fabro et al., 2001; Griffits et al., 2003), and consequently that it is important to describe its components, other authors question the need for such calculation (Silva & Gomez, 2009).There are also researchers such as Chung et al., (1997) who prefer to report the components in concentrations and absolute quantities. Nevertheless, Znahg et al., (2002) and Griffiths (2003) stated that the correct interpretation of results is dependent on the volume of GCF collected.

Evaporation is considered to be a technical difficulty particularly affecting small volumes (Tozum et al., 2004). However, intervals up to 30 seconds between sample collection and volume measurement do not interfere with measurements.

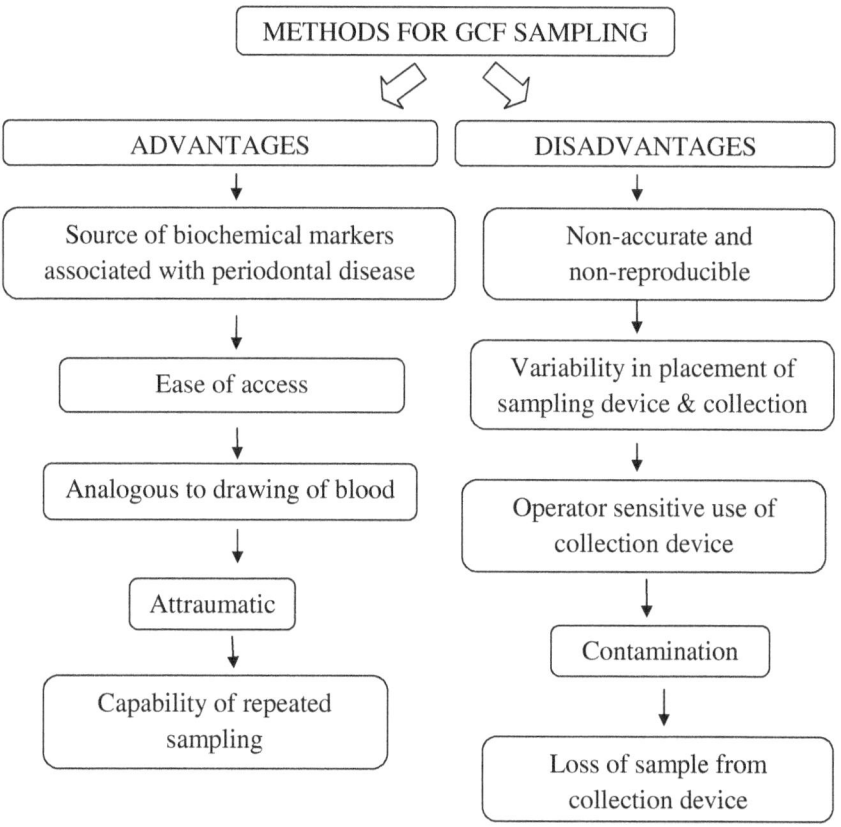

Figure 5. General advantages and disadvantages of GCF sampling methods

Gingival crevicular fluid (GCF) is a marker of periodontal inflammatory condition as well as periodontal healing. Collecting the initial GCF by absorbent paper strips offers a possibility of rapid measurement of its volume and composition thus decreasing the probability of altering the GCF by excessive contamination with serum (Tzannetou et al., 1999).

General advantages and disadvantages of the GCF sampling methods are shown in Fig. 5.

5. THERAPEUTIC APPROACHES IN PERIODONTAL DISEASE

Periodontal diseases are the most common dental conditions. They begin as an infection; however they appear to behave not like classic infection but more like an opportunistic infection. This fact that periodontal disease contains a microbial and inflammatory component makes it extremely difficult to treat (Ryan, 2005).

Periodontal therapies can be divided into three broad categories:

- Mechanical debridgement and cleaning to eliminate the bacteria, a procedure also known as scaling and root planning (SRP) ;
- Mechanical treatment (SRP) combined with addition of certain chemotherapeutic agents such as systemically or locally applied antimicrobials or antiseptics
- Mechanical treatment (SRP) combined with the so called "host-modulatory agents" which affect the environment of the infectious microorganisms.

Scaling and root planning (SRP) is a non-surgical traditional treatment modality for periodontitis that focuses on reduction of the total bacterial count in the periodontal pockets. This non-specific treatment has proven successful on a long term basis for many patients, although a small but relevant proportion of the patients may not respond adequately (Drisko, 2001). In certain cases, bacterial deposits in deep pockets are difficult to remove and may be responsible for the poor treatment outcome of SRP alone.

The adjunctive use of systemic or locally applied antibiotics may provide additional periodontal benefit over SRP alone, but this treatment is not without side effects or adverse reactions attributed to the antibiotic. Systemic antibiotics are of particular benefit in combating severe forms of periodontal disease such as aggressive periodontitis and necrotizing periodontitis

(Slots & Ting, 2002). The primary candidates for systemic antibiotic therapy are patients who exhibit continuous periodontal breakdown and alveolar bone loss despite mechanical debridgement. In cases where systemic drug application seems inappropriate, local delivery formulations are of particular use. Local application of antimicrobials especially benefits patients suffering from localized periodontitis (Horz and Conrads, 2007). The principal therapeutic benefit of a localized periodontal delivery is that it can selectively target therapy to the sites most requiriring additional treatment (Galler, 2005).

Advances in the understanding of periodontal etiology as well as clinical data obtained from current research have shown that periodontal tissue destruction is a complex result of bacterial biofilm, bacterial enzymes and toxins and the host's response to them (Oringer, 2002). It has become evident that host-derived inflammatory mediators such as matrix metalloproteinases (MMPs), cytokines and other inflammatory molecules such as PGE_2 are responsible for the majority of tissue destruction in the periodontium.

This shift has led to the development of the so called Host Modulatory Therapies (HMT), which can improve therapeutic outcomes, slow the progression of the disease, allow for more predictable management of patients and possibly even work as preventive agents against the development of periodontits (Thompson, 2001; Reddy et al, 2011). In the last two decades scientists have investigated various host modulating strategies in both animal and human experimental models. Up to date, specific aspects considered for modulation of periodontitis pathogenesis include:
- regulation of production of arachidonic acid metabolites
- regulation of bone remodeling
- regulation of matrix metalloproteinase (MMPs) activity.

The host modulatory agent group consists of nonsteroidal anti-inflammatory drugs (NSAIDs), biphosphonates, matrix metalloproteinase activity inhibitors and corticosteroids.

5.1 Corticosteroids as therapeutic modality in periodontal disease

Glucocorticosteroids drugs are synthetic analogues of hormones and these substances are used to suppress inflammation in a wide variety of diseases including allergic diseases, rheumatoid arthritis, inflammatory bowel disease and autoimmune diseases (Barnes, 1998). They have been used in every aspect of oral medicine due to their potent anti-inflammatory and immunosuppressant properties (Savage &McCullogh, 2005).

The anti-inflammatory action of corticosteroids is based on a range of actions involving glucocorticoid receptors, the glucocorticoid responsive genes, and the release of anti-inflammatory molecules such as lipocortin-1, interleukins Il-10, Il-1 and nuclear factor-kB by macrophages, eosinophills, lymphocytes, dendritic cells, neutrophills and endothelial and epithelial cells. The anti-inflammatory molecule lipocortin-1, a member of annexin super-family of proteins, is one of the "second messengers" of anti- inflammatory action of glucocorticoids, acting through inhibition of prostaglandin formation as well as playing a major regulatory role in systems such as cell growth regulation and differentiation, neutrophil migration, CNS response to cytokines, neuroendocrine secretion, and neurodegeneration. Glucocorticoids also induce the transcription of the gene, encoding the inhibitor of factor Kappa B subtype a (IkBa), which reduces the amount of NF-kB that translocates to the nucleus and the secretion of pro-inflammatory cytokines. The immunosuppressant effect of corticosteroids is derived mainly from the suppression of antigen-driven T-cell proliferation through the inhibition of interleukin-1release from monocytes. At higher doses, they can also interfere with antibody formation. Corticosteroids can, therefore, reduce the migration of leukocytes and exudation of plasma constituents, thereby eliminating the edema and maintaining the integrity of cell membranes. They also help avoid the excessive swelling of cells, inhibit the release of lysozymes from granulocytes and phagocytosis, and stabilize the membrane of the intracellular lysosomes, thereby avoiding the further release of hydrolytic enzymes, intracellular digestation, and spread of the inflammatory process. Corticosteroids also inhibit fibroblast proliferation suppressing fibrosis (Ghanbachi et al., 2009).

Corticosteroids can be applied either locally or systemically in the treatment of different conditions in oral pathology and periodontology. Several animal studies have confirmed that systemically administered steroids have adverse effects on the periodontium and its response to bacterial plaque (Seymour, 2006). Experimental studies have demonstrated that the use of systemic corticosteroids can provoke many conditions on the periodontium ranging from gingival ulceration to the down migration of the epithelium, attachment loss and disruption of transseptal fibers. In addition, systemic use of high doses of glucocorticosteroids leads to inhibition of fibroblast activity, loss of collagen and connective tissue with decreased reepithelisation and angiogenesis, reduction in the number and activity of osteoblasts and increased osteoclast function (Garcia et al., 2010).

The frequency and severity of the adverse effects associated with the use of systemic corticosteroids have led to the increased use of topical corticosteroids. Topically, their predominant anti-inflammatory action appears to be on prostaglandin formation, edema inhibition and stabilizing the lysosomal membranes, thus suppressing the release of lytic enzymes (Fachin et al., 2009).

Topical corticosteroids can be divided into several categories as a function of their potency. The most commonly used topical corticosteroids on oral pathology are given in Table 1. In general, mild and moderate topical corticosteroids are used for long term treatments while potent and very potent products are preferred for shorter regimens.

Table 1. *Synthetic topical corticosteroids used in oral pathology*

Potency	Dose % (w/w)	Topical corticosteroid
Mild		Hydrocortisone
	1	Hydrocortisone acetate
	0.25	Methylprednisolone
	0.05	Alclometasone dipropionate
	0.01-0.1	Dexamethasone
	0.0025	Fluocinolone acetonide
	0.75	Fluocortin butyl ester
	0.5	Prednisolone
Moderate	0.05	Clobetasone butyrate
	0.02	Triamcinolone acetonide
	0.005	Fluocinolone acetonide
Potent	0.05	Betamethasone dipropionate
	0.1	Betamethasone valerate
	0.025	Fluocinolone acetonide
	0.1	Hydrocortisone butyrate
	0.05	Halomethasone monohydrate
	0.1	Diflucortolone valerate
Very potent	0.1	Halcinonide
	0.05	Clobethasol propionate

Conventional dosage forms of topical corticosteroids include creams, ointments, lotions or gels.

According to our knowledge, there are only few studies that address the effect of locally applied corticosteroids on periodontal healing. When these molecules are injected directly into the gingival tissue, they cause a histological reduction in capillary permeability, a reduction in plasma cells and granulation tissue, an inhibition of collagen synthesis and a clinical improvement in hemmoragic and hypoplastic gingivitis (Safkan and Knuuttila, 1984). However, current research data suggest that locally applied corticosteroids show favorable effects on periodontal healing and possess anti-resorbtive effects. Dexamethasone directly affects osteoclast formation and activity, stimulating the proliferation and differentiation of human osteoclast precursors, and inhibiting the bone resorbtion activity in mature osteoclasts (Hirayama et al., 2002). Teeth treated with 0.05% clobetasol and 0.05% fluocinonide show favourable periodontal healing; the higher potency corticosteroid clobetasol exerts more favorable healing than the lower potency fluocinonide. It remains unclear whether the antiresorbtive effect of these compounds can be further enhanced by using corticosteroid with increased potency and its anti-inflammatory properties. Although concern exists that the use of corticosteroids locally in the periodontium may induce hypothalamus-pituitary-adrenal axis, it has been reported that the highest possible amounts used are unlikely to result in any systemic side effect (Kirakozova et al., 2009). The chemical structures of several synthetic topical corticosteroids used in oral pathology are given in Fig. 6.

While topical application of corticosteroids for skin disorders is well documented, there is considerably less critical information available for lesions of the oral mucosa, including periodontal disease.

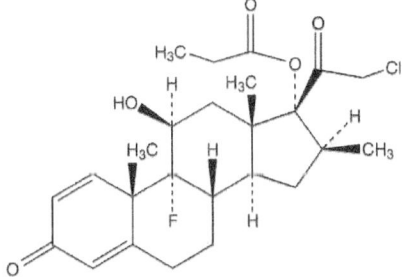

Figure 6. Synthetic corticosteroids used topically in the oral cavity for various inflammatory disorders

Having in mind that the character of the vehicle system defines the potency of the topical preparation and its selection its critical for product performance, it can be concluded that there is a need for further research into therapeutic systems that improve local delivery of corticosteroids to oral mucosa and periodontium as well as controlled clinical studies in order to evaluate the clinical effectiveness of these formulations attended for treatment of periodontal lesions.

5.2. Betamethasone dipropionate as adjunct to periodontal treatment

Betamethasone dipropionate (BDP) is a semi-synthetic, fluorinated, highly potent glucocorticoid receptor agonist designed to exert marked glucocorticoid activity and finds widespread clinical application related to its anti-inflammatory, anti-proliferative and immunosuppressive activity (Pereira et al., 2005). It is frequently used in everyday clinical praxis as an adjunct to scaling and root planning as well as in the tretatment of lesions of the oral mucosa. It exerts its action by inhibition of phospholipase A_2 which leads to the inhibition of arachidonic acid synthesis and controls the biosynthesis of prostaglandins and leukotriens (Fachin et al., 2009). There are various types of dosage forms for BDP such as ointment, cream, lotion and foam which are primarily used in the treatment of mild to moderate inflammatory skin disorders including psoriasis (Dyderski et al., 2002). Compared to other corticosteroids intended for local application on periodontal tissues, such as hydrocortisone or triamcinolone acetonide, BDP shows greater anti-inflammatory action probably due to stabilization of lysosomal membranes and blocking the actions of the invasive mediators of inflammation (Fachin et al., 2009).

5.3 Methods for the analysis of corticosteroid molecules in biological samples

Corticosteroids comprise a large group of natural substances that must be frequently monitored in various biological samples because they regulate many aspects of the metabolism and the immune function. Additionally, numerous synthetic steroids have been used as therapeutic agents in the treatment of various disease (Shimada et al., 2001).

The qualitative and quantitative of steroids, including corticosteroids in biological matrices such as human body fluids or animal tissues is not trivial. Their structures are closely similar and they contain several functional groups, which in most cases can make their separation quite difficult. Furthermore, corticosteroids can be metabolized in peripheral or target tissues to gain or lose their biological activity (Pacha et al., 2004).

In order to analyze the impact of natural and synthetic steroids on the organism, there is an urgent need for good analytical techniques capable to determine the individual compounds of interest. These techniques should be not only sensitive but also selective. This means that one needs not only to determine low concentrations of corticosteroids in biological samples (can be a considerable problem) but also to separate individual steroids of interest and to separate these steroids from other accompanying compounds of different chemical nature (Makin et al., 1995; Shimada et al., 2001; Shu et al., 2003).

A review of the literature has shown that corticosteroids in various biological samples can be identified and quantified by several analytical techniques. The analysis can be performed by using immunoassays, gas chromatography coupled to mass spectrometry or liquid chromatography.

Immunoassays provide rapid analysis but suffer from several serious disadvantages. They have low assay specificity, inadequate standardization and poor optimization of the method over the large range of concentrations seen clinically (Middle, 1998; Thienpont, 1998). The lack of sensitivity often makes these systems unsuitable for clinical applications that require a low detection limit. The cross-reactivity as well as the necessity to use many different types of kits to cover the wide range of corticosteroids are additional problems related to the application of these techniques in routine laboratory analysis.

Gas chromatography-mass spectrometry (GC-MS) is a valuable method used to analyse the metabolites of steroid hormones and their precursors, especially in urine. GC-MS will continuously play an active role in studying rare and undefined conditions and retains its place as the pre-eminent discovery tool for defining new and aberrant metabolic pathways and for first-time characterization of unknown steroids (Krone et al., 2010). In spite of these advances, several drawbacks limit its application in routine analysis. GC-MS methods require long analysis times and time consuming derivatisation in order to visualize and quantify the analyte of interest in the complex biological matrix.

Liquid chromatography (LC) is widely used for separation and determination of various substances in different matrices. Compounds that differ in their molecular properties, like hydrophobicity, polarity and ionic character can be separated and analysed without prior derivatisation with the large number of techniques that LC offers.

Reversed-phase high performance liquid chromatography (RP-HPLC) is an advanced form of liquid chromatography and a refinement of traditional column chromatographic techniques. Due to its high degree of sensitivity and selectivity, it's one of the most commonly used tools in the quantitative analysis of small molecules in different types of samples.

RP-HPLC can be routinely employed in everyday clinical praxis and it is attractive because of the simplicity of sample processing and high-throughput put. The speed of analysis and the resolution are increased with new column packaging materials and eluants through the column at high pressures. One of the mostly used detectors in HPLC is the UV detector which is capable of monitoring several wavelengths concurrently. The potential for monitoring concentrations of steroids in small volume samples is limited both in physiological and pathological conditions. Using HPLC-UV, the detection limit can be only a nanogram per milliliter sample (Honour, 2006). However, the right sample treatment procedure must be carefully chosen in order not to cause high interference from the sample matrix.

Although RP-HPLC has certain disadvantages such as high initial investment and the cost of chromatographic columns, the overall possibilities presented by this technique have made HPLC one of the most important techniques for chromatographic analysis of corticosteroids. The advantages of application of HPLC in corticosteroid analysis include (Honour, 2006):

- short time for chromatographic analysis (few minutes per sample)
- high temperatures are not required
- wide choice of stationary and mobile phases for optimal separation
- full recovery of column eluates for further analytical procedures
- superior resolution compared to that of TLC or paper chromatography
- potential and versatility for separation of intact conjugates
- although most steroids can be quantified by HPLC-UV, their metabolites lack UV chromophores and can be detected using refractive index detector or electrochemical detector

- possibility to find more information from spectra when using diode array detector
- possibility of coupling HPLC to mass spectrometers
- automatisation leading to higher productivity

5.4 RP-HPLC methods in periodontal therapeutic drug monitoring

Therapeutic drug monitoring (TDM) is the measurement of drugs and their metabolites for the purpose of optimizing their therapeutic effects while minimizing adverse effects. In general, biological specimens most frequently used in TDM are plasma, serum, urine, and nowadays, saliva.

Clinical parameters traditionally used to monitor periodontal treatment include probing depths, bleeding on probing, clinical attachment levels, plaque index, and radiographs assessing alveolar bone level. The strengths of these traditional tools are their ease of use, their cost-effectiveness, and the fact that they are relatively noninvasive. Unfortunately, traditional diagnostic procedures are inherently limited, in that only disease history, not current disease status, can be assessed (Armitage, 2004).

Among clinical investigators in periodontology, clinical studies that test the effectiveness of chemotherapeutic agents are of special interest. Drugs that are excreted through the gingival fluid may be used advantageously in periodontal therapy.

Studies for localized drug delivery for targeted release of the therapeutic agent in the periodontal pocket are of increasing frequency. The GCF formed in the periodontal pockets provides a reservoir for certain drugs that enter the pocket through the systemic circulation. Also, the GCF provides a leaching medium for drugs applied locally in the periodontal pocket and at the same time GCF enables drug distribution throughout the pocket (Jain et al. 2008). Furthermore, advances in the etiology, epidemiology and microbiology of the periodontal disease have shown that certain drugs frequently used in periodontal treatment have a unique ability to concentrate in gingival tissues and GCF because gingival fibroblasts serve as their reservoirs. Clinical studies have shown that doxycycline, metronidazole and ciprofloxacin concentrate in gingival fibroblasts (Lavda et al., 2004; Agnihotri et al., 2012; Tomasi et al., 2011).

The efficacy of chemotherapeutic agents in periodontitis cannot be evaluated using the traditional clinical parametars and cannot reflect the therapeutic concentrations the drug achieves in GCF. Knowing the advantages of RP-HPLC such as high sensitivity and precision for measuring concentrations in small volume samples such as GCF, the conclusion derived is that it can be used for monitoring the therapeutic concentration of drugs used to treat periodontitis.

Having in mind that GCF represents a unique window for monitoring periodontal conditions and drug concentrations in periodontal pockets, sensitive RP-HPLC methods for routine clinical application may serve for therapeutic drug monitoring and optimizing individual treatment in periodontitis patients.

6. AIM OF THE STUDY

After the introduction of topical corticosteroid formulations, their use has become widespread for treating large variety of dermatological conditions as well as different inflammatory lesions of the oral mucosa. Topical application of drug dosage forms to the tissues of the oral cavity is used as an essential part in the treatment of toothache, periodontal diseases, bacterial and fungal infections aphtae and stomatitis (Brushi & Freitas, 2005).

Betamethasone dipropionate cream 0.5 mg g^{-1} is applied routinely as adjunct to scaling and root planning. It's potent topical anti inflammatory and host's modulatory activity shows great potential in the local periodontal treatment given to patients suffering from localized forms of periodontal disease.

The applied BDP cream 0.5 mg g^{-1} is a conventional dosage form and has short residence time in periodontal pockets. Although it shows favorable effects on periodontal healing, one might say that as a conventional dosage form, the cream may be unsuitable for application in the periodontal pockets.

Having in regard that GCF can serve as a valuable reservoir for drugs used in the periodontal treatment, it might be important to determine how much of the applied dose of BDP enters the fluid using the advantages of the HPLC methodology.

According to our knowledge, no HPLC method for determination of BDP concentration in GCF could be found in literature, while some RP HPLC and HPLC-MS methods have been developed for determination of BDP in biological samples.

Hence, the goals of our research arose:

- Development and optimization of a bioanalytical RP-HPLC method with UV detection for determination of betamethasone dipropionate in gingival crevicular fluid ;
- Validation of the optimized RP-HPLC method as per EMEA guideline ;
- Application of the developed and validated bioanalytical RP-HPLC method for determination of BDP in GCF samples taken from periodontitis patients treated with local application of BDP cream 0.5 mg g^{-1} ;
- Investigation of the concentrations of BDP in GCF after the application of 0.05 % BDP cream.

7. MATERIALS AND METHODS

7.1 Materials
1. Betamethasone dipropionate working standard, Farmabios, Italy
2. Alclomethasone dipropionate working standard (internal standard, IS), Crystalpharma (Spain)
3. BELODERM® cream 0.5 mg g^{-1}, BELUPO
4. Whatman 3MM chromatography paper strips 2 x 5 mm, Whatman Lab Sales Ltd., UK

7.2 Gingival crevicular fluid (GCF) samples

GCF samples were obtained from patients attending the Department of Periodontology, Faculty of Dentistry, Skopje.

7.3 Human serum samples
Human serum was obtained from healthy volunteers from the Faculty of Dentistry, Skopje.

7.4 Chemical and reagents
1. Water HPLC grade, TKA–LAB Reinstwasser system
2. Methanol HPLC grade, Merck, Germany
3. Potassium dihydrogen phosphate, analytical grade, Fluka, Switzerland.

7.5 Instrumentation
1. Mechanical vortex, Heidolph, REA, Germany
2. Analytical balance, Sartorius, Germany
3. HPLC analysis

All experiments were performed on the Agilent 1100 HPLC system equipped with vacuum degasser (G1322A Degasser), a quaternary pump (G1311AQuatPump), auto sampler (G1313A ALS), a column compartment

(G1316A COLCOM), diode array detector (G1315B DAD) and ChemStation for LC 3D software for data handling (Wilmington, DE).

7.6 Chromatographic conditions

The chromatographic separation was performed on C18 analytical column (Purospher STAR RP 18-e 120 Å, 150 x 4.6 mm, 5-µm), using LiChroCART® 4-4 guard column (Merck, Germany). The HPLC system was maintained at 25°C with MeOH:0.04 mol L^{-1} KH_2PO_4 (70:30, V/V) as mobile phase. The flow rate was 1.3 mL min^{-1}. The mobile phase was filtered through 0.45 µm cellulose membrane filter (Millipore, Bedford, MA, USA) prior use. The injection volume was 100 µL. UV detection was performed at 245 nm. The total run time for the HPLC analysis was 14 min.

7.7 Collection of GCF samples

GCF samples were obtained from fifty patients suffering from localized periodontitis at the end of the periodontal treatment (one week after the beginning of the scaling and root planinig procedure). Quadrants consisting of 5 teeth were treated with 0.1 mL 0.5 mg g^{-1} BDP cream containing 27 µg betamethasone dipropionate (BELODERM® cream 0.5 mg g^{-1}, BELUPO), using blunt needle. Samples for analysis were taken 15 minutes after treatment. Patients were in good general health and had not taken any antibiotic or anti-inflammatory drug in the previous three months. The procedure was approved by the Ethical Committee of Faculty of Dentistry, University of Ss. Cyril and Methodius, Skopje. GCF was collected applying the method of Koss et al. (Koss et al., 2009) and taken by placing 2 x 5-mm Whatman paper strips into the pocket (depth 4-6 mm) until mild resistance was felt and left there for 30 s. Strips contaminated with blood were excluded from analysis.

7.8 Preparation of standard solutions and quality control (QC) samples

Stock standard solutions of betamethasone dipropionate (1.00 mg mL^{-1}) and alclomethasone dipropionate (1.00 mg mL^{-1}) were prepared in methanol and refrigerated at 4 °C. Working standard solutions of BDP were made daily by diluting the stock standard solution of BDP with mobile phase to concentrations of 50.00, 125.00, 250.00, 375.00 and 500.00 μg mL^{-1}, respectively. Working standard solution of IS was made daily by diluting the stock standard solution of IS with mobile phase to concentrations of 100.00 μg mL^{-1}. Calculations were performed assuming a volume of one μL GCF (based on the volume that could be collected in the periodontal pocket and which is consistent with dental practitioner experience).

Calibration curve standard solutions were prepared using working standard solutions of BDP and IS on six paper strips previously spiked with 1 μL of serum, in the following manner: One μL of separate BDP working standard solution was added to separate paper strip, then 10 μL of IS working standard solution was added to each paper strip. Paper strips were extracted with 500 μL MeOH:H$_2$O mixture (70:30, *V/V*). Final concentrations of calibration curve standard solutions were 0.10, 0.25, 0.50, 0.75, 1.00 and 2.00 μg mL^{-1}.

QC samples were prepared in the same manner as calibration curve standard solutions in concentrations of 0.10, 0.25, 1.00 and 1.75 μg mL^{-1} and stored at -20 °C. GCF exists as a serum transudate, therefore QC samples and calibration curve standard solutions were prepared in serum because GCF is not commercially available nor easily collectable in large volumes (Vinneay & Kindberg, 1997).

7.9 GCF sample preparation

After collection of GCF, paper strips were removed and placed in preweighted Eppendorf tubes and kept at -20 °C until analysis. Before the

HPLC analysis, GCF samples were thawed at room temperature. 10 μL from 100 μg mL^{-1} IS solution was added to the GCF sample. After adding a mixture of methanol/water (70:30, V/V) as an extracting solvent up to volume of 500 μL, the GCF sample solutions were vortex mixed for 3 minutes. The liquid content of the tubes was transferred to glass autosampler vials. A 100-μL aliquot was injected into the chromatographic system. The weight of the fluid was calculated from the differences between masses of the strips with GCF and dry strips. The obtained value, expressed as μg, was converted to volume in μL assuming the density of GCF was 1 mg mL^{-1} (Koss et al., 2009). The whole process for GCF sample preparation is shown in Fig. 7.

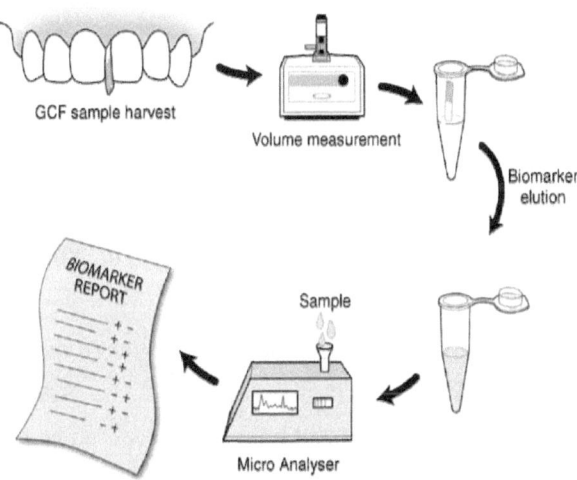

Figure 7. GCF sample preparation process

7.10   Bioanalytical method validation

Method validation was conducted according to the Guideline on Validation of Bioanalytical Methods of the European Medicines Agency (EMEA, 2009).

The main characteristics of the bioanalytical method essential to ensure the acceptability of performance and the reliability of results are the following:

Selectivity

Selectivity was assessed by comparing the chromatograms of blank GCF samples from six sources and those obtained from GCF spiked with the analyte(s) of interest and internal standard.

Linearity and range

Prior to validation of the bioanalytical method, the concentration range should be justified based on scientific information. The range should be covered by the calibration line range, defined by the lower limit of quantification (LLOQ) and the upper limit of quantification (ULOQ). A minimum of six calibration concentration levels should be used, excluding blank sample (processed matrix sample without analyte and IS) and zero sample (processed matrix with IS). The acceptable criterion for each standard concentration should be ±15 % of the nominal concentration, except for LLOQ which is ±20 %.

Accuracy and precision

Accuracy and precision were assessed on samples spiked with known amounts of analyte, the quality control samples (QC samples). Accuracy and precision were evaluated for the values of the QC samples obtained within a single run (the with-in run) and in different runs (the between-run). With-in run accuracy and precision were determined in at least five samples per concentration level on LLOQ, low, medium and high QC samples in a single run.

Between-run accuracy and precision were assessed by five determinations per concentration per run on LLOQ, low, medium and high QC samples from three runs analysed on at least two different days.

Accuracy was expressed as a mean percent deviation (RE) of the observed concentration (c_{obs}) from the nominal concentration (c_{nom}) at each concentration level using the following formula:

$$\% \text{ RE} = [(c_{obs} - c_{nom})/ c_{nom}] \times 100$$

Precision was calculated as the percent of coefficient of variation (% CV, % RSD) by the following formula:

$$\% \text{ CV} = (SD/\text{mean } c_{obs}) \times 100$$

% CV determined at each concentration level should not exceed 15%, except for LLOQ where it should not exceed 20%.

Recovery

Recovery describes the efficiency of the extraction procedure used in the analytical process. The extraction recovery for BDP and the IS were calculated by comparing peak areas measured after extraction of five replicates of LLOQ, low, medium and high QC with peak areas of solutions with same concentration prepared in the mobile phase which served as standards.

% Recovery = (BDP peak area $_{samples}$)/ (BDP peak area $_{standards}$) x 100

Stability

For the purpose of bioanalytical method validation, the stability of the stock standard solutions of BDP and IS and the stability of BDP in the sample matrix was examined. Stability tests were performed under setting likely to be encountered during sample collection, storage, preparation and analysis. BDP sample solution stability was tested by chromatographic analysis of QC samples at LQC and HQC levels. The freeze-thaw stability (36 h at - 20 °C, three cycles), short-term stability (2h, room temperature, 25 °C ± 2 °C), long-term stability (14 days, -20 °C) and autosampler stability (immediately after extraction and 16 hours after preparation) were investigated.

The stability of the stock solutions should be evaluated at room temperature for at least 6 hours. For this evaluation, stock solutions of BDP and IS were prepared. Each stock solution was divided into two parts. One half was stored at room temperature (20-25 °C) for 7 days and the other half was stored under refrigeration (2-8 °C). All solutions were kept protected from light during the stability testing period.

8. RESULTS AND DISCUSSION

Betamethasone dipropionate is a potent semi-synthetic topical corticosteroid with anti-inflammatory and immune-suppressive properties. Conventional pharmaceutical dosage forms of BDP include creams, ointments, aerosols, injectables and lotions. It can be combined with salicylic acid, tolnaftate or calciprotriene in the treatment of corticosteroid-responsive dermatoses (Vairale et al., 2012).

The extent of percutaneous absorption of topical BDP is determined by many factors including the vehicle, the integrity of the epidermal/mucosal barrier and in some cases the occlusive dressings. BDP can be absorbed through normal, intact skin. Inflammation or other disease processes in the skin or oral mucosa can increase the percutaneous absorption. Once absorbed, it enters pharmacokinetic pathways similar to systemically administered corticosteroids. It is bound to plasma proteins in varying degrees; it's metabolized primarily through the liver and excreted through the urine. Local and systemic adverse effects are rare, ranging from local irritation to reversible hypothalamic-pituitary-adrenal (HPA) axis suppression. Betamethasone dipropionate has seventeen known potential degradation products and process related impurities (Kaur et al., 2010). When applied topically BDP reaches low concentrations in the body, which makes its analysis in biological samples a special challenge.

Most chromatographic techniques that are used for separation and determination of BDP in biological and other types of samples have been developed for simultaneous determination of BDP with other molecules. A literature search has shown several methods for determination of BDP in pharmaceutical formulations (Kaur et al., 2010; Shou et al., 2009). An LC-MS method for quantification of BDP in human plasma was developed as discussed by Zou (Zou et al., 2008) in order to assess the pharmacokinetics of betamethasone phosphate/betamethasone dipropionate injection in healthy Chinese volunteers. Other methods for the analysis of BDP include GC-MS and LC-MS analysis in animal tissues and waste waters.

Bioanalytical methods are a set of all procedures involved in the collection, processing, storing and analysis of the biological matrix for an analyte (Shah et al., 1992). Analytical methods employed for the qualitative and quantitative determination of drugs and their metabolites in various biological samples are the key determinants in generating reproducible and reliable data that in turn are used in the evaluation and interpretation of bioavailability, bioequivalency and pharmacokinetics (Shah et al., 2000).

The LC-MS methods have been widely applied techniques in the analysis of various biological samples that are highly selective and sensitive. In this way, tandem mass spectrometry looks very attractive for the analysis of different types of steroids, and often require little sample pretreatment. Although mass spectrometric detection could be the method of choice for many corticosteroid analyses, it is not suitable for routine use in many laboratories, mainly in developing countries. These techniques require highly trained personnel and the cost of such approach as well as the expertise needed may lower against its routine use (Makin et, al., 1995).

The HPLC-UV methods offer substantial selectivity and sensitivity and can be routinely used in laboratory praxis. These methods can be successfully used for qualitative and quantitative monitoring of drugs such as corticosteroids excreted in the gingival crevicular fluid.

An RP-HPLC method for determination and quantification of betamethasone dipropionate was developed and optimized. The impact of several chromatographic parametars such as mobile phase composition, buffer concentration and flow rate was examined. In addition, special attention was given to the sample pretreatment procedure.

8.1 Optimization of a RP-HPLC method for determination of BDP in GCF

8.1.1 Considerations for the method development

Analytical method development is the process of creating a procedure to enable a compound of interest to be identified and quantified in a matrix. A compound can often be measured by several methods and the choice of analytical method involves many considerations, such as: chemical properties of the analyte, concentrations levels, sample matrix, cost of the analysis, speed of the analysis, quantitative or qualitative measurement, precision required and necessary equipment. The analytical chain describes the process of method development and includes sampling, sample preparation, separation, detection and evaluation of the results.

Betamethasone dipropionate is chemically 9-fluoro-11β,17,21-trihydroxy-16β-methylpregna-1,4-diene-3,20-dione 17,21-dipropionate, with the empirical formula $C_{28}H_{37}FO_7$, molecular weight of 504.59. From the chemical structure of this compound it appears that there aren't any functional groups that can be easily ionized. Therefore, mobile phase pH and ionic strength should not affect the retention or the separation of the molecule under RP-HPLC conditions (Xiao et al., 2008, Kaur et al., 2010). Hence, in our study, these parameters were not optimized or evaluated during method development.

In this case method development and optimization should be focused on the selection of suitable selection of the RP-HPLC analytical column, optimization of the mobile phase composition, selection of the most suitable wavelength and optimization of the sample pretreatment procedure. Although, the analyte retention time should change as a function of the column temperature, the practical usable temperature range is not very wide for methods that are intended for routine use.

The column selection should be based on the surface properties of the stationary phases and the properties of the analyte. Having in mind that corticosteroids are hydrophobic molecules, typically they can be analyzed using traditional hydrophobic reverse phase packing, such as C18 packing. C18 stationary phases have been reported to give excellent peak shapes and offer appropriate resolution for detection and quantification of corticosteroid molecules such as betamethasone dipropionate. Thus a simple C18 analytical column can be used because it's stable and rugged.

The commonly used organic solvents in RP-HPLC are methanol (MeOH), acetonitrile (ACN), and to a lesser extent ispropanol and tetrahydrofuran (THF). For the separation of corticosteroid molecules in biological samples, binary mobile phases usually consisting of methanol/acetonitrile with water/buffers such as potassium dihydrogen phosphate have been used. In our study we chose MEOH to be the organic solvent and potassium dihydrogen phosphate as the buffer solution. MeOH was favoured as the organic solvent because it resulted in well separated, sharp peaks of the analyte and internal standard. MeOH has higher viscosity compared to ACN, which can lead to higher column back pressure and problems operating the HPLC system but has lower cost than ACN. However, higher column back pressure was not evident in our study. Optimization of various parameters was performed in order to develop a sensitive and selective HPLC method with UV detection for analysis of BDP in human GCF. A KH_2PO_4 buffer based mobile phase was first investigated to develop a fully validated assay method using UV detection.

8.1.2 Identification of BDP and IS in GCF sample

Identification of BDP was achieved by chromatography of standard substances dissolved in MeOH or mobile phase under the same conditions as biological samples and comparing the retention times observed.

8.1.3 Optimization of the mobile phase composition and flow rate

During the preliminary investigations, the mobile phase composition and flow rate of the mobile phase were optimized. Several mobile phases containing buffer 0.04 mol L^{-1} KH_2PO_4 and methanol were investigated where the composition of the organic phase varied from 60-80% (organic phase/buffer, V/V). In the beginning, 35% 0.04 mol L^{-1} KH_2PO_4 and 65% MeOH (V/V) was set to be the initial mobile phase. This resulted in inacceptable retention time for the BDP molecule. Having in mind that a higher proportion of organic solvent increased the mobile phase strength and reduced the retention time of the analyte, it was not surprising that the mobile phase composition of 25% 0.04 mol L^{-1} KH_2PO_4 and 75% MeOH gave faster retention time for BDP. Due to the fact that the latter mobile phase composition was less economical and still the best result was obtained using mobile phase containing 30% 0.04 mol L^{-1} KH_2PO_4 and 70% methanol (V/V), this was set as the final mobile phase. The composition of the mobile phase was also adjusted to eliminate the interferences from blank GCF.

Optimization of the mobile phase flow rate was also performed. Three flow rates were investigated and the BDP peak area and retention time were compared. The flow rate was investigated in the range from 0.8-2 mL min^{-1} and the final flow rate was set at 1.3 mL min^{-1}. This flow rate was chosen as the optimal to aid in the reduction of the overall runtime yet still having an acceptable column back pressure.

8.1.4 Selection of suitable wavelength of detection

As shown in literature, steroid compounds, including BDP, are determined using wavelengths at which the analyzed compounds exhibit absorption maxima. The mostly used wavelength for detection is 254 nm (Qi et al., 2008). Preliminary investigations for the optimal wavelength of detection were performed with the working standard solutions containing 500 µg mL^{-1} BDP and internal standard, alclomethasone dipropionate. Knowing that BDP achieves low concentrations in biological matrices, such as GCF, further experiments were conducted with spiked GCF samples containing 0.10 µg mL^{-1} BDP (LLOQ). The UV absorbance spectrum of BDP under the applied conditions contained an absorbance maximum at 245 nm. Finally, the wavelength of 245 nm was selected for detection.

8.1.5 Optimization of the buffer concentration

Potassium dihydrogen phosphate buffer was tested by varying its concentration at 0.01 mol L^{-1}, 0.025 mol L^{-1}, 0.04 mol L^{-1}, 0.075 mol L^{-1} and 0.10 mol L^{-1}. Increasing buffer molarity above 0.04 mol L^{-1} did not result in any significant changes in the chromatographic response and peak symmetry, so this buffer was selected for further analysis (Fig. 8).

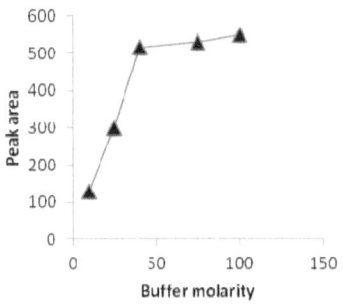

Figure 8. Peak area versus buffer molarity plot

8.1.6 Optimization of the injection volume

In order to achieve the required accuracy, precision and sensitivity for selective determination of BDP in GCF several injection volumes were tested. The injected sample volume was varied between 20-100 µL. It was found that 100 µL was optimal to obtain maximum peak enhancement especially for the extracted samples in which the lowest concentration of BDP was expected.

8.1.7 Selection of the column temperature

The column temperature was set at 25 °C because the BDP molecule and the internal standard could be adequately separated.

8.1.8 Selection of the internal standard

The proper selection of an internal standard is of great importance in the development of a biomedical method. Current giudelines for bioanalytical method validation recommend the usage of internal standards, which are a good marker for extraction recovery and the quality of the chromatographic procedure.

The most favourable characteristics of the ideal internal standard include: it should be completely resolved from all the peaks in the sample, it should elute near the sample, it must behave similarly to the analyte in the pretereatment of the samples so that losses could be correlated (Lehrer, 2010). In this way, the internal standard could also be used for estimating the overall extraction recovery.

In our study, we used alclomethasone dipropionate as an internal standard. Alclomethasone dipropionate has very similar structure (Fig. 9) and elutes near to BDP. Furthefmore, it showed an acceptable retention time, absorbtivity and a symetrical peak. Alclomethasone dipropionate elutes without having interferences with any of the components of the matrix (GCF sample without BDP) and therefore fulfills the requirements to be used as an internal standard in the chromatographic analysis.

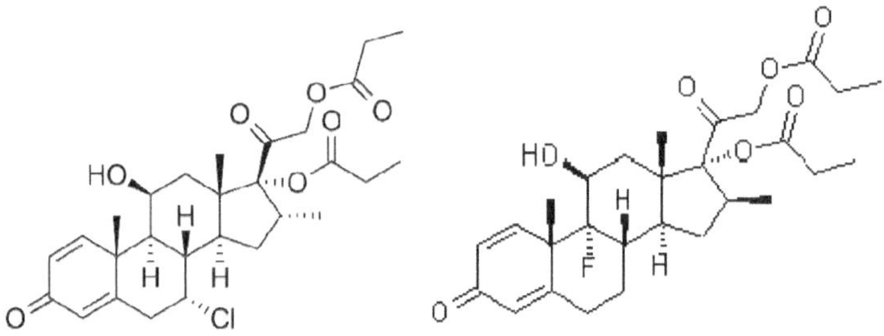

Figure 9. Chemical structure of alclomethasone dipropionate (a) and BDP (b)

After all of these method optimizations, the retention times for BDP and the IS were 11.01 and 6.5 min, respectively. The total run time for each analysis was set at 14 min. The optimal chromatographic conditions are shown in Table 2.

Table 2. *Optimized chromatographic conditions for determination of BDP in GCF*

Parameter	Optimized conditions
Analytical column	Purospher STAR RP 18-e, 150 x 4.6 mm i.d.; 5μM
Mobile phase	Solvent A methanol 70%
	Solvent B potassium dihydrogen phosphate 0,04 M 30%
Flow rate	1,3 ml/min
Column temperature	25°C
Detection wavelength	245 nm
Injection volume	100μl

8.1.9 Optimization of the sample pretreatment procedure for determination of BDP in GCF samples

Good sample preparation is often the key to successful analytical results. It has a direct impact on accuracy, precision and quantification limits and is often the rate determining step for many analytical methods. The purpose of sample preparation is to clean up the sample before analysis and/or to concentrate the sample. Material in biological samples that can interfere with analysis, the chromatographic column or the detector includes proteins, salts, endogenous macromolecules, small molecules and metabolic byproducts. Injection of matrix substances can also cover up and hide the drug or analyte being analyzed, making quantification difficult or even impossible. A goal with the sample preparation is also to exchange the analyte from the biological matrix into a solvent suitable for injection into the chromatographic system.

BDP is reported to be very soluble in MEOH, ACN, acetone, isopropanol or tetrahydrofuran. Based on this information, some preliminary experiments were carried out pointing to the use of MeOH/water as the extracting solvent. Hence, the use of different ratios of MeOH/water were explored. The optimization of various sample preparation/extraction parameters were performed using blank GCF samples. All these experiments were conducted in order to assess the influence of different extraction steps on the recovery of the analyte, BDP and the recovery of the IS molecule.

The total protein content in GCF samples is much less than serum (Patel, 2011), thus samples were injected directly into the HPLC system. However, the pre-analytical treatment of GCF samples was essential to obtain cleaner extracts.

The following sample preparation/extraction parameters were tested: (i) variation of the amount of MeOH in the extraction solvent (different MeOH/water ratios), (ii) variation of the vortex time and (iii) premixed versus non-premixed extraction solvent. We did not test filtered versus non filtered solutions since GCF contains small amount of proteins and we inject approximately only 1 µl of GCF sample.

After testing all the conditions, a premixed MeOH/water (70:30, V/V) as the extracting solvent and 3 minutes vortex time was the best combination for sample extraction. By using these extraction conditions and procedure, full recovery of BDP and IS from GCF was obtained.

8.2 Bioanalytical method validation

The main objective of method validation is to demonstrate the reliability of a particular method for the determination of an analyte concentration in a specific biological matrix, such as plasma, serum, urine, saliva, different tissues or GCF. All applied bioanalytical methods must be well characterized, fully validated and documented to a satisfactory standard in order to yield reliable results (EMEA, 2009).

Each validation batch contained the following samples:
- Extracts from calibration curve standards to obtain the calibration line
- Extracts of quality control samples to assess the accuracy and the precision of the method
- Extracts of blank GCF samples to which no internal standard has been added to monitor the possible carryover from previous injections and for the possible appearance of other interfering peaks
- Extracts of zero samples which are GCF extracts to which no internal standard was added

The parameters investigated during method validation were: linearity, selectivity, intra- and inter-day accuracy and precision, analyte recovery and stability.

8.2.1 Selectivity

Method selectivity is the ability of an analytical method to produce a response for the target analyte, distinguishing it from all other components present in the analyzed sample. The selectivity was investigated by comparing blank GCF sample solutions and QC sample solution containing 0.10 µg mL^{-1} BDP. In order to evaluate any possible exogenous interference, chromatograms from the mobile phase were also compared. Since the patients enrolled in the study did not take any medications that concentrate in GCF and gingival tissues, we did not expect interferences from other drugs in the matrix. Representative chromatograms of the mobile phase, blank GCF samples and GCF samples spiked with 0.10 µg mL^{-1} BDP are shown in Fig. 10, Fig. 11 and Fig 12, respectively.

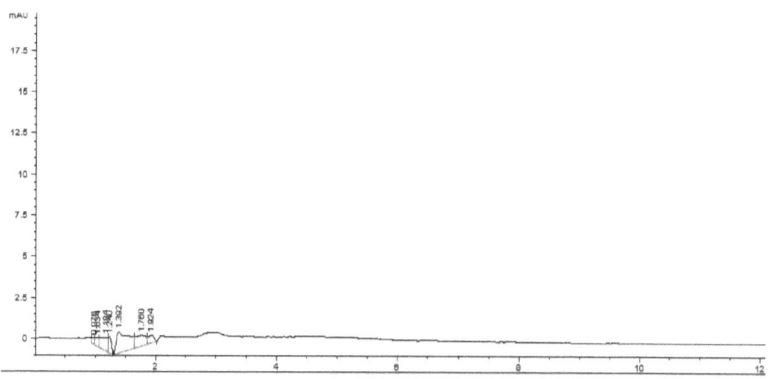

Figure 10. Chromatogram of the mobile phase

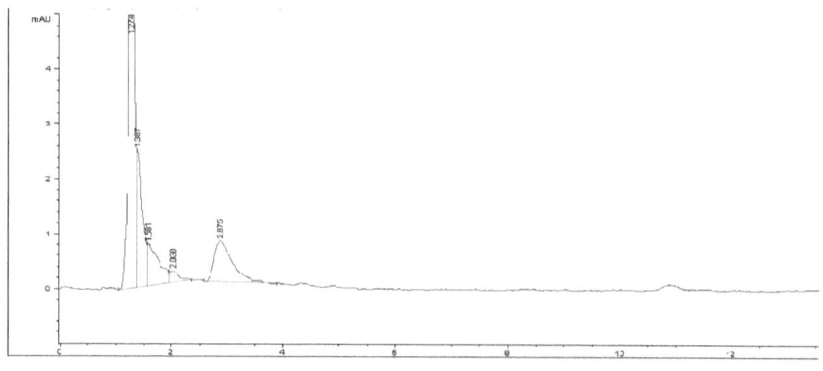

Figure 11. Representative chromatogram of a blank GCF sample

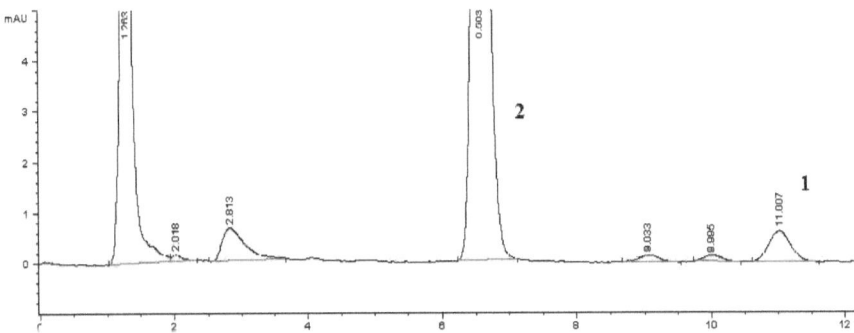

Figure 12. Representative chromatogram of a QC sample containing 0.10 µg mL^{-1} BDP (1) and 2.00 µg mL^{-1} IS (2).

As shown in Fig. 12, BDP and the IS were well separated under the applied HPLC conditions and resolved with good symmetry. The retention times for BDP and IS were 11.01 min and 6.5 min, respectively. No endogenous interfering peaks at the retention times of BDP and IS were observed in the mobile phase and in blank GCF samples, confirming the selectivity of the method.

8.2.2 Linearity

A six point calibration curve, in the range of 0.10-2.00 µg mL^{-1} BDP in GCF, including LLOQ and ULOQ was constructed. The concentration range for the calibration curve was that expected in the final extracted GCF sample injected on the column. The calibration curve was obtained using linear regression analysis of BDP peak area to IS peak area ration vs. concentration. Limit of detection (LOD) was calculated as the concentration level resulting in peak area three times the baseline noise, while lower limit of quantification (LLOQ) was calculated as analyte response area at least five times the blank response. Analyte calculated concentration at the LLOQ level should be reproducible with the precision ≤ 20 % and accuracy of 80-120 %.

Good linearity with high determination coefficient (R^2= 0.9971) was observed by plotting peak area ratios of BDP and IS against the BDP concentrations over the examined concentration ranges. LOD was 0,05 µg mL^{-1} and LLOQ was 0,10 µg mL^{-1}. Important calibration curve parameters: slope (a), intersept (b), coefficient of determination (R^2), as well as limit of detection (LOD) and limit of quantification (LOQ) are given in Table 3.

Table 3. *Calibration curve parameters*

Parametar	Obtained value
a±SD	-0,003 ±0,0356
b±SD	0,513 ±0,0036
R^2	0,9971
LD	0,05 µg mL^{-1}
LLOQ	0,10 µg mL^{-1}

8.2.3 Accuracy and precision

Intra-day (with-in run) and inter-day (between–run) accuracy and precision were determined using five replicates of each of the following QC sample solutions: 0.10, 0.25, 1.00 and 1.75 µg mL^{-1} which represent lower limit of quantification (LLOQ), low QC sample (LQC), medium QC sample (MQC) and high QC samples (HQC) respectively. Chromatograms of LQC samples and HQC sample are shown in Fig. 13 and Fig. 14, respectively.

Table 4. *Intra-day and inter-day accuracy and precision*

	BDP in QC sample ($\mu g\ mL^{-1}$)[a]	Found concentration ($\mu g\ mL^{-1}$)[a]	Accuracy (%)[b]	Precision (RSD, %)
Intra-day	0.100	0.109±0.004	109.6	3.5
	0.250	0.246±0.009	99.7	4.0
	1.000	0.967±0.025	96.6	2.2
	1.750	1.728±0.078	98.7	4.5
Inter-day	0.100	0.106±0.152	106.0	4.4
	0.250	0.247±4.651	99.1	3.3
	1.000	0.969±2.231	97.0	1.6
	1.750	1.767±0.101	101.0	5.7

[a] Each sample solution contains 2.00 $\mu g\ mL^{-1}$ IS.
[b] Mean±SD, n=5

The relative standard deviations (intra-day and inter-day) and obtained values for accuracy are presented in Table 4. As it can be seen from the results, intra-day precision ranged from 2.2-4.5% and intra-day accuracy ranged from 98.7-109.6%. Inter-day precision and accuracy ranged from 1.6-5.7 % and 97.0-106.0 %, respectively.

In conclusion, all the values obtained for accuracy and precision are within limits regarded as acceptable for the analysis of biological samples (85-115%).

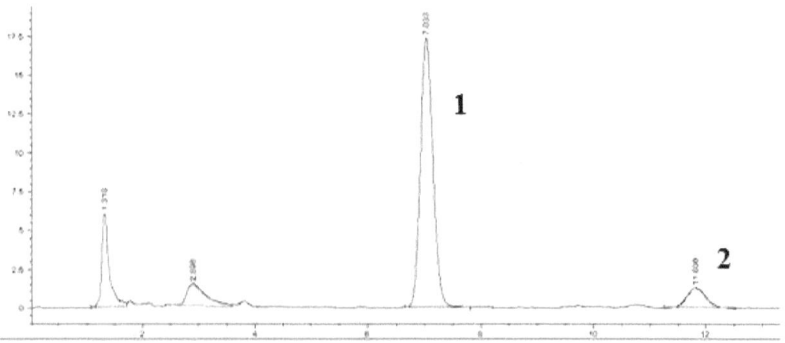

Figure 13. Representative chromatogram of LQC sample containing 0.25 µg mL^{-1} BDP (1) and 2.00 µg mL^{-1} IS (2).

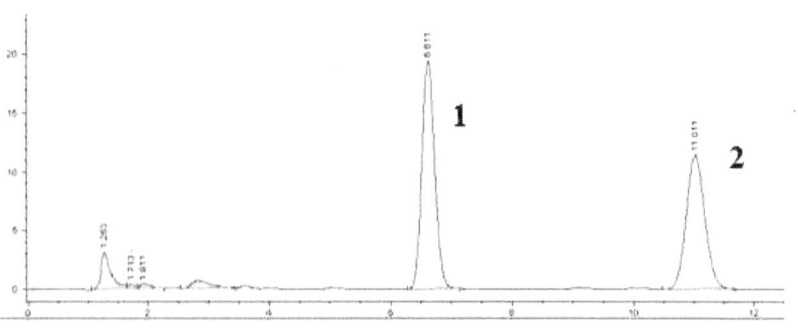

Figure 14. Representative chromatogram of HQC sample containing 1.75 µg mL^{-1} BDP (1) and 2.00 µg mL^{-1} IS (2).

8.2.4 Recovery

In analytical chemistry the main goal is to determine the identity and/or concentration of one or more species in a sample. Therefore, the extraction procedure must result in a satisfactory recovery of both the analyte and the internal standard.

The mean extraction recovery of BDP from the matrix at four concentration levels (0.10, 0.25, 1.00 and 1.75 µg mL^{-1}) were 87.9, 99.6, 101.0 and 99.5%, respectively. The obtained extraction recovery values that are higher than 100% are likely due to the preparation process. The recovery for the internal standard, alclomethasone dipropionate, was 98.2%. The results are presented in Table 5.

Table 5. *Extraction recovery data*

Concentration of BDP in QC sample solutions (µg mL^{-1})	Recovery (%)[a]	RSD (%)[b]
0.10	87.9	2.90
0.25	99.6	7.89
1.00	101.0	0.32
1.75	99.5	0.26
Internal standard (µg mL^{-1})		
2.00	98.2	3.02

[a] Expressed as mean peak area ratio of extracted samples/mean peak area ratio of the unextracted samples
[b] Expressed as RSD: (SD/mean) x 100

The recovery of BDP from the matrix, using the described procedure, was consistent and efficient.

8.2.5 Stability

Drug stability in a biological fluid is a function of the storage conditions, the chemical properties of the drug, the matrix, and the container system.

The stability of the analyte should be established preferably prior to sample analysis. Stability procedures should evaluate the stability of the analytes during sample collection and handling, after long-term (frozen at the intended storage temperature) and short-term (bench top, room temperature) storage, and after going through freeze and thaw cycles and the analytical process.

Stock solution of BDP and IS were stable at room temperature for 24 h (recovery: 99.5 and 99.8%, respectively) and at 2 – 8 °C for one month (recovery: 99.1 and 98.5%, respectively). Under both, room temperature and refrigerated conditions, relative difference was within ± 5% of the initial concentration. No additional peaks were observed at any time points in comparison to day 0 of analysis.

The results showed that GCF samples spiked with BDP are stable after three freeze-thaw cycles, after 16 hours in the autosampler and at room temperature for 2 hours. The study also indicated that samples could be kept frozen at -20 °C for two weeks. The results are presented in Table 6.

8.2.6 Analysis of patient GCF samples

In order to investigate the potential of the validated method for clinical studies, it was applied to determine the BDP concentrations in GCF samples obtained from patients with localized chronic periodontitis after the local treatment with BDP 0.5 mg g^{-1} cream. After the HPLC analysis, considering all the steps in extraction and sample preparation procedures, BDP concentration was calculated and then expressed per mL of collected sample. The obtained values for BDP concentrations are shown in Table 7. Representative chromatograms of patient GCF sample are shown in Fig. 15 and Fig. 16.

Table 6. *Stability data for betamethasone in GCF samples*

Storage condition	BDP in QC sample ($\mu g\ mL^{-1}$)	Determined BDP (%)[a]	
		Fresh samples ($\mu g\ mL^{-1}$)	% relative to fresh samples
Freeze-thaw stability	0.100	0.099 ± 0.005	99.0 ± 3.5
	1.750	1.726 ± 0.004	99.0 ± 0.4
Short-term stability	0.100	0.100 ± 0.001	100.3 ± 2.0
	1.750	1.722 ± 0.001	98.6 ± 0.4
Autosampler stability	0.100	0.102 ± 0.002	101.2 ± 0.7
	1.750	1.732 ± 0.003	98.0 ± 2.0
Long-term stability	0.100	0.101 ± 0.004	101.0 ± 3.9
	1.750	1.737 ± 0.010	99.7 ± 0.7

[a] Mean±SD, n=5

All included patients completed the study and BDP was quantified in all measured samples. No adverse reaction was observed in any subject from the test group and no patient reported any discomfort. All subjects tolerated well the drug without any post application complications. As it can be seen from Table 6, the concentrations of BDP in the analyzed GCF samples varied in the range 0.10-1.80 µg mL^{-1} per collected sample. The variability of the concentrations of BDP in human GCF samples is probably a result of different pocket depth, as assumed by Tsai et al., (Tsai et al., 1998) and Goodson (Goodson, 2003) that deeper periodontal pockets contain larger volumes of excreted GCF.

BDP has been used extensively in the control and treatment of periodontal disease as adjunct to the non-surgical treatment. Conventional pharmaceutical dosage forms of BDP include cream and ointment. In order to avoid the contact with the oral mucosa, BDP cream is applied subgingivally in the inflamed periodontal pocket. Creams seem to be more suitable for application in periodontal pockets, due to the moist environment in the oral cavity (Dyderski et al., 2002). Following topical application, BDP produces potent anti-inflammatory, vasoconstrictive and immunosuppressive action thus local drug delivery of immuno-modulatory agents can down regulate the disease without the need of subjecting the entire body to unnecessary exposure of the drug. The concentrations of BDP in GCF were examined in our study.

Overall, using the specific, sensitive and validated HPLC method, our findings indicated that BDP is released from the cream and penetrates well in GCF. As potent corticosteroids, such as BDP are used frequently in periodontal treatment, the penetration of the active compound in GCF during the increased secretion induced by the disease itself may be the key factor in the effectiveness of the therapy.

The flow rate of GCF can differ several times between normal periodontium and patients with periodontitis. It is possible that the diffusion process of active compounds from topically applied dosage forms into crevicular fluid depends on the flow rate. Repeated collection of GCF can cause gingival tissue irritation, which in turn can influence the flow rate

(Goodson, 2003). The high flow rate can be the reason for fast evacuation of the already released drug in the periodontal pocket to the surrounding tissues, thereby depleting the effective concentration of the chemotherapeutic agent in the periodontal pocket. On the one hand, one limitation of this study might be the single time point for sample collection after drug application. However, the sample collection time is consistent with the fact that topical preparations containing potent corticosteroids should be applied 10-15 min at most.

One of the limitations of this study might be the relatively small number of patients included. Factors related to the immune response of each individual may have a strong impact on the therapy outcome. Therefore, a larger sample group would provide more information about the efficacy of the BDP topical therapy.

The low concentrations of BDP in GCF after the local application may be due to unsuitable dosage form and rapid release of BDP in GCF, which is typical for conventional dosage forms. New treatment strategies are directed towards developing new cream or gel formulations with improved mucoadhesive properties that might provide more sustained/controlled delivery of the chemotherapeutic agent in the periodontal pocket.

Periodontal pockets may be used as natural sites for easy placement of micro/nanoparticulate delivery systems (Alvarez et al., 2011). Systems that contain natural biopolymers, such as chitosan and alginate micro/nanoparticulate systems may overcome the limitations of the short-time release profile of conventional dosage forms used in the treatment of periodontitis.

Table 7. *BDP concentrations in periodontitis patients after the local periodontal treatment with BDP cream 0.5 mg g^{-1}*

Patient №	BDP concentration (µg ml^{-1})	Patient №	BDP concentration (µg ml^{-1})
1	0.62	26	0.95
2	0.45	27	0.47
3	0.59	28	0.31
4	0.42	29	0.32
5	1.71	30	0.66
6	0.66	31	0.36
7	0.55	32	0.29
8	0.98	33	0.31
9	0.72	34	0.69
10	1.64	35	0.47
11	1.03	36	1.80
12	0.35	37	0.49
13	0.28	38	0.98
14	1.25	39	1.71
15	0.51	40	0.26
16	0.71	41	1.81
17	0.57	42	0.10
18	1.03	43	1.24
19	0.10	44	0.15
20	1.19	45	0.57
21	1.47	46	0.67
22	0.10	47	0.14
23	0.57	48	0.59
24	0.46	49	1.00
25	0.14	50	0.69

Successful periodontal therapy depends on establishing and monitoring effective drug concentrations of the anti-inflammatory agent at the diseased site. Considering significant inter-individual variability in BDP concentrations in GCF among patients after the local periodontal treatment, there is a potential clinical relevance of therapeutic drug monitoring in order to find the optimal therapeutic regimen. The proposed method is suitable for use as a standard method for analysis of BDP in GCF for future products and product modifications for the treatment of periodontal disease.

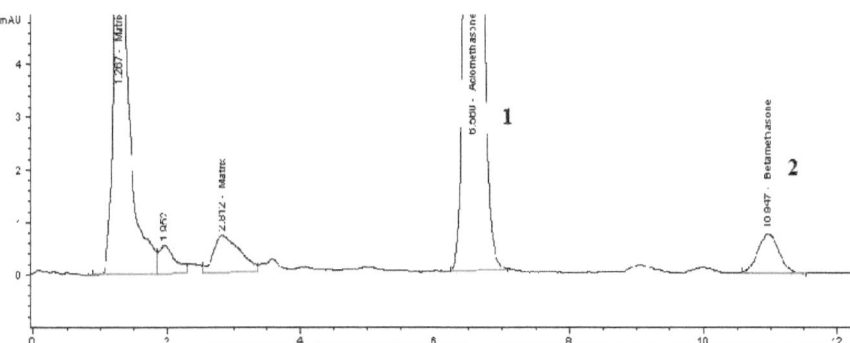

Figure 15. Representative chromatogram of a patient's GCF sample obtained after the local periodontal treatment with 0.5 mg mL^{-1} BDP cream. The sample contains 2.00 µg mL^{-1} IS (1) and 0.10 µg mL^{-1} BDP (2). Unnamed peaks are endogenous components from the matrix.

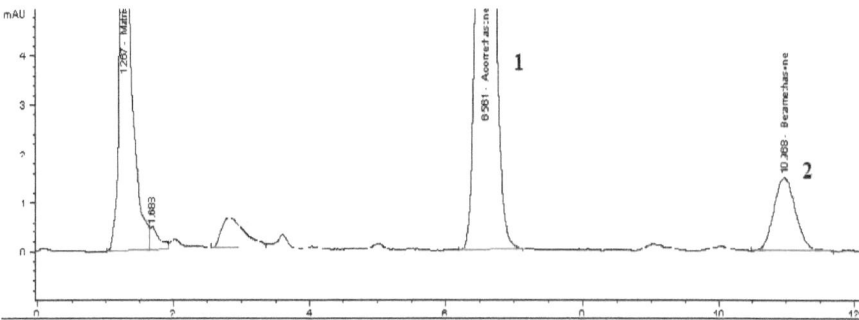

Figure 16. Representative chromatogram of a patient's GCF sample obtained after the local periodontal treatment with 0.5 mg mL^{-1} BDP cream. The sample contains 2.00 µg/mL IS (1) and 0.25 µg mL^{-1} BDP (2). Unnamed peaks are endogenous components from the matrix.

9. CONCLUSION

Researchers involved in delivering periodontal therapy are currently investigating the possible use of oral fluids such as GCF and saliva in diagnosis, drug development and therapeutic drug monitoring. Determination of effective concentrations of drugs used in periodontal treatment using instrumental techniques such as HPLC may be used as a therapeutic approach leading towards individualized therapy.

- In our study, an isocratic bioanalytical RP-HPLC method with UV detection for determination of BDP in GCF samples has been optimized, developed and validated ;

- The method optimization systematically investigated the crucial chromatographic parameters: mobile phase composition, wavelength of detection, flow rate, selection of a suitable stationary phase, buffer concentration and injection volume. Alclomethasone dipropionate was used as internal standard. The optimization procedure resulted in the following method characteristics: a stable and rugged C_{18} stationary phase was chosen, the mobile phase consisted of MeOH and KH_2PO_4 (70:30, v/v) and the flow rate was set at 1.3 ml/min. The analyte of interest and the IS were detected at 245 nm and the injection volume was 100 μL ;

- The sample preparation procedure for extraction of BDP from GCF samples was simple and efficient. The optimized extraction procedure was easy, using MeOH/water (70/30, v/v) as extraction solvent. Analyte loss was fully avoided, no sample concentration, solvent evaporation and reconstitution steps yielded high values of recoveries with small degree of variations ;

- Validation of the optimized bioanalytical RP-HPLC method was conducted in accordance with the Guideline on Validation of Bioanalytical methods of the European Medicines Agency:

➢ Under the optimized chromatographic conditions the BDP peak was well separated from the components of the matrix. No interfering peaks from the matrix and no exogenous interferences from the mobile phase appeared at the retention of BDP or IS, and thus the selectivity of the method was confirmed ;

➢ Linearity was observed in the range 0.10-2.00 µg mL^{-1}, LOD was 0.05 µg mL^{-1} and LLOQ was 0.10 µg mL^{-1}. The high value for the correlation coefficient (R^2 = 0.9971) obtained for the developed method indicated that the proposed method is linear, and the values obtained for the LLOQ show that the method is sensitive ;

➢ The obtained values for intra-day accuracy and precision ranging from 98.7-109.6% and 2.2-4.5% and results for inter-day accuracy and precision 97.0-106.0% and 1.6-5.7% show that the proposed bioanalytical method is accurate and precise ;

➢ The values for the mean extraction recovery for BDP at four concentration levels ranged from 87.9-101.0, and the recovery for the internal standard was 98.2%. The dependence on concentration was negligible. The sample preparation was simple and yielded satisfactory values for the recovery ;

- The stability experiments aimed at testing all the possible conditions that the samples might experience between collection and analysis showed that GCF samples spiked with BDP are stable after three freeze-thaw cycles, after 16 hours in the autosampler, at room temperature and should be kept frozen at – 20 °C for two weeks ;

- The optimized and validated method was applied to the analysis of BDP in human GCF samples taken from patients after the local periodontal treatment with BDP cream 0.5 mg g^{-1}. Considering high sensitivity and small aliquots of biological sample needed for analysis, this method can be easily applied to other pharmacokinetic and distribution studies from similar dosage form which contain BDP as the active ingredient ;

- Our study indicates that BDP penetrates well into GCF. The main advantage of the present study was the use of patients without any induction of GCF flow and the use of sensitive, specific and validated HPLC method ;

- The significant inter-individual variability in BDP concentrations among patients found in our work suggest that there is a potential clinical relevance of the therapeutic drug monitoring of BDP in GCF in order to find the optimal therapeutic dose regimen ;

The proposed method has a number of advantages such as high sensitivity and separation efficacy, simple mobile phase and low price of chromatographic columns. The short run time decreases the solvent consumption, thus providing economic benefit. Recently, analytical methods of liquid chromatography/tandem mass spectrometry have been established for measuring BDP concentrations in biological samples. They demonstrate excellent sensitivity but involve complicated sample preparation procedures, demand higher expense for instrument maintenance and highly trained personnel.

Thus, our established analytical method with UV detection is suitable for routine measurement of BDP in GCF. As a result of all the mentioned advantages, this method can find its application in the analysis of clinical samples in order to plan the proper type and extent of periodontal treatment.

10. REFERENCE

Agnihotri R., Gaur.G., Chemically modified tetracyclines: novel therapeutic agents in the management of chronic periodontitis, Ind. J. Pharmacol. 44: 161-167 (2012)

Albandar J. M., Global risk factors and risk indicators for periodontal disease, Periodontol. 2000. 29: 177-206 (2002)

Alvarez L. A., Espinar O. F., Mendez B. J., The application of microencapsulation techniques in the treatment of endodontic and periodontal diseases, Pharmaceutics. 3: 538-571 (2011)

Aras H., Çaglayan F., Güncü G. N., Berberoğlu A. and Kilinc K., Effect of systematically administered naproxen sodium on clinical parametars and myeloperoxidase and elastase – like activity levels in gingival crevicular fluid, J. Periodontol. 78: 868-873 (2007)

Armitage C.G., The complete periodontal examination, Periodontol. 2000. 34: 22–33 (2004)

Attin T., Mbiydzemo F. N., Villard I., Kielbassa A. M., Hellwig E., Dental status of Schoolchildren from a rural community in Cameron, J. S. Afr. Dent. Assoc. 54: 145-148 (1999)

Barnes J. P., Anti-inflammatory actions of glucocorticoids: molecular mechanisms, Clin. Sci. 94: 557–572 (1998)

Berezov A. and Darveau R., Microbial shift and periodontits, Periodontol 2000. 55(1): 36-47 (2011)

Brushi M. L., Freitas O., Oral bioadhesive drug delivery system, Drug Dev. Ind. Pharm. 31: 293-310 (2005)

Champagne C., Buchanan W., Reddy M., Preisser J., Beck J., Offenbacher S., Potential for gingival crevice fluid measures as predictors of risk for periodontal diseases, Periodontol 2000. 31: 167-180 (2003)

Ciantar M., Caruana D.J., Periotron 8000: Calibration characteristics and reliability. J. Period. Res. 33:259-264 (1998)

Del Fabro, Francetti L., Bulfamante G., Cribiu M., Misserocchi G., Weinstein R.L., Fluid dynamics of gingival tissues in transition from physiological condition to inflammation, J. Periodontol. 72: 65-73 (2001)

Deinzer R., Mossanen B.S., Herforth A., Methodological considerations in the assessment of gingival crevicular fluid volume, J. Clin. Periodontol. 27: 481-488 (2000)

Dincel A., Yildirim A., Caglayan F., Bozkurt A., Determination of ciprofloxacin in human gingival crevicular fluid by high-performance liquid chromatography, Acta Chrom. 15 :308-314 (2005)

Drisko H. C., Non surgical periodontal therapy, Periodontol. 2000. 25: 77-88 (2001)

Dyderski S., Grzeskoviak E., Szalek E., Mrzyglod A., Pharmaceutical availability of betamethasone dipropionate and gentamicin sulfat from cream and ointment, Acta Pol. Pharm. 59 (2): 99-103 (2002)

Fachin E., Scarparo R., Pezzi A., Luisi S., Filho M., Effect of betamethasone on the pulp after topical application to the dentin of rat teeth: vascular aspects of inflammation, J. Appl. Oral Sci. 17(4): 335-339 (2009).

Fachin E., Zaki A., Hystology and lysosomal cytochemisty of the postsurgically inflamed dental pulp after topical application of steroids. Histological study, J. Endo. 9: 457-460 (1991).

Garsia V., Fernandes L., Almeida J., Bosho F., Nagata M., Martins T., Okamoto T., Theodoro L., Comparison between laser therapy and non-surgical therapy for periodontitis in rats treated with dexamethasone, Lasers. Med. Sci. 25(2): 197-206 (2009).

Giannopolou C., Kamma J.J., Mombelli A., Effect of inflammation, smoking and on gingival crevicular fluid, J. Clin. Periodontol. 30: 145-53 (2003)

Guideline on validation of bioanalytical methods, European Medicines Agency, Committee for Medicinal Products for Human Use (CHMP), London; http://www.ema.europa.eu/docs/en_GB/document_library/Scientific_guideline/2009/12/WC500018062.pdf. (2009)

Ghanbachi J., Najafi R., Hagnegahdar S., Treatment of oral inflammatory with a new mucoadhesive prednisolone tablet versus triamcinilone acetonide paste, Iran. Red Cres. Med. J. 11(2):155-159 (2009).

Griffits G., Formation, collection and significance of gingival crevice fluid. Periodontology 2000. 31:32-42 (2003)

Goodson J. M., Gingival crevice fluid flow, Periodontol. 2000. 31:43-45 (2003)

Figueredo C.M.S, Gustafson A., Protease activity in gingival crevicular fluid, J. Clin. Periodontol. 25: 306-310 (1998)

Hamasha A.A., Sasa I., Al-Qudah M., Risk indicators asstiated with tooth loss in Jordanian adults, Community Dent. Oral Epidemiol. 28: 67-72 (2000)

Hanioka T., Matsuse R., Shigemoto Y., Ojima M., Schzukuishi S., Relationship between periodontal disease status and combination of biochemical assays of gingival crevicular fluid, J. Periodon. Res. 40: 331-338 (2005)

Horz H. & Conrads G, Diagnosis and antiinfective therapy of periodontitis, Exp. Rev. Antiinfect. Ther. 5(4): 703-715 (2007).

Honour J., High performance liquid chromatography for hormone assay in Methods in molecular biology. 324:25-52 Wheeler M., Hutchinson J. (Edit.), Humana press Inc., Totowa NJ (2006).

Hirayama T., Sabokbar A., Athanasou A.N., Effect of corticosteroids on human osteoclast formation and activity, J Endo. 175: 155-163 (2002)

Jain N., Gaurav K., Shamama J., Zeenat I., Sushama T., Farhan J. A., Roop K. K., Recent approaches for the treatment of periodontitis, Drug Disc. Tod, 13: 932-942 (2008)

Johnson R. B., Streckfus C. F., Dai X., Tucci M.A., Protein recovery from several paper types used to collect gingival fluid, J. Periodon. Res. 34: 283-289 (1999)

Kantarci K., Van Dyke T., Lipoxin signaling and their role in periodontal disease, Prosta. Leukotr, Ess. 73: 289-299 (2005)

Kavadia-Tsatala S., Kaklamanos E., Tsalikis L., Effects of orthodontic treatment on gingival crevicular fluid flow rate and composition: Clinical implications and applications, Int. J. Adult Orthodont. 17(3): 191-205 (2002).

Kaur P., Wilmer G, Wei Y, Rustum A.M., Development of a stability-indicating RP-LC method for determination of betamethasone dipropionate and estimation of its related compounds in a dermatological pharmaceutical product, Chromatographia. 9(10): 805-814 (2010).

Kinney J., Ramseier C., and Giannobile W., Oral Fluid-based Biomarkers of Alveolar Bone Loss in Periodontitis, Ann.N.Y. Acad Sci. 1098: 230-251 (2007).

Kirakozova A., Texeira F., Curran A., Gu F., Tawil P., Trope M., Effect of intracanal corticosteroids on healing of replanted dog teeth after extended dry times, J Appl End. 35: 663-667 (2009)

Kirkwood K., Cirreli J., Rogers J., Giannobile W., Novel host response therapeutic approaches to treat periodontal diseases, Periodontol. 2000. 43: 294-315 (2007).

Kornman S. K., Page R.C., Tonneti S. M., The host response to the microbial challenge in periodontitis: assembling the players, Periodontol. 2000. 14: 33-53 (1997)

Koss M., Castro S., Lopez M., Enzimatic Profile of Gingival Crevicular Fluid in Association With Periodontal Status, Lab. Med. 40 (5): 277-280 (2009).

Krone N., Hughes B., Lavery G., Stewart P., Arlt W., Shackleton, Gas chromatography/mass spectrometry (GC/MS) remains a pre-eminent discovery tool in clinical steroid investigations even in the era of fast liquid chromatography tandem mass spectrometry (LC/MS/MS), J. Steroid. Biochem. Mol. Biol. 121(3-5): 496–504 (2010)

Lavda M., Clausnitzer E.C., Walters D.J., Distribution of systemic ciprofloxacin and doxycyline to gingival and gingival crevicular fluid, J. Periodontol. 75: 1663-1667 (2004)

Lehrer M., Chromatographic techniques. In Kaplan L.A., Pesce A.J., (Edit.). Clinical chemistry: Theory, analysis and correlation. 5th Ed., St. Louis (MO): Mosby, p: 84(2010)

Liew V., Mack G., Tseng P., Cvejic M., Hayden M., Buchanan N. Single dose concentrations of tinidazole in gingival crevicular fluid, serum and gingival tissue in adults with periodontitis, J. Dent. Res. 70(5):910-912 (1991).

Linden G.J., Mullally B.H., Burden D.J., Lamey P.J., Shaw C., Ardill J., Changes in vasoactive intestinal peptide in gingival crevicular fluid in response to periodontal treatments, J. Clin. Periodontol. 29: 484-489 (2002)

Loos B. & Tjoa S., Host-derived diagnostic markers for periodontitis, Periodontol 2000. 39:53-72 (2005).

Makin H.L.J., Gower D.B., Kirk D. N., Steroid analysis, Blackie, London. p: 204-225 (1995)

Malamud D. and Rodriguez-Chavez I., Saliva as a diagnostic fluid, Dent Clin North Am. 55 (1): 159-178, 2011.

Malhotra R., Grover V., Kapoor A., Kapur R., Alkaline phosphatase as a periodontal disease marker, Ind. J. Dent Res. 21(4): 531-536 (2010).

Middle J, Standardization of steroid hormone assays, Ann Clin Biochem. 35:354-363 (1998)

Offenbacher S., Periodontal diseases: pathogenesis, Ann. Periodontol. 1 (1): 821-878 (1996)

Oringer J. R., Modulation of the host response in periodontal therapy. J. Periodontol. 3: 460-70 (2002)

Ozkavaf A., Aras H., Huri C.B., Yamalik N., Kilinc A., Kilinc K., Analysis of factors that may affect the enzymatic profile of gingival crevicular fluid: sampling technique, sequential sampling and mode of data presentation, J. Oral. Sci. 43: 41-48 (2001)

Patel V. P., Gingival crevicular fluid (GCF). an oral biomarker in the diagnosis and quantification of periodontal diseases, J. Invest. Periodontol. 3(6): 45-63 (2010)

Pácha J., Mikšik I., Mrnka L., Zemanová A., Brindová J., Mazanková K., Kučka M. Cortocosteroid regulation of colonic ion transport during postnatal development : Methods for corticosteroid analysis. Physiolog. Res. 53(1): 63-80 (2004).

Pähkla E-R, Koopel T, Saag M, Pähkla R., Metronidazole concentrations in plasma, saliva, and periodontal pockets in patients with periodontitis, J. Clin. Periodontol. 32: 163-166 (2005).

Pereira S.A., Oliveira L., Mendes G., Gabbai J., Nucci G., Quantification of betamethasone in human plasma by liquid chromatography-tandem mass spectrometry using atmospheric pressure photoionisation in negative mode, J. Chrom. B. 828: 27-32 (2005)

Qi X. H., Simultaneous determination of nandrolone, testosterone, and methyltestosterone by multi-immunoaffinity column and capillary electrophoresis, Electrophoresis. 29: 3398-3405 (2008)

Reddy Shapira. Essentials of Clinical Periodontology and Periodontics. 2nd Edition. Jaypee Brothers, Medical Publishers, Reddy, India (2008).

Reddy S., Prasad M.GS., Kaul S., Asutkar H., Bhowmik N., Host modulation in periodontics. E-J Dent., 1: 51-62 (2011)

Ryan M. E., Nonsurgical approaches for the treatment of periodontal disease, Dent. Clin. North Amer. 49: 611-636 (2005)

Savage W.N., McCullogh J.M., Topical corticosteroids in dental practice, Aust Dent J. 50: 40-44 (2005)

Safkan, B., Knuuttila, M., Corticosteroid therapy and periodontal disease, J. Clin. Periodontol. 11: 515-522 (1984)

Serra E., Perrinetti G., Attilio M. D', Cordella C., Paolantonio M., Festa F., Spoto G., Lactate dehydrogenase activity in gingival crevicular fluid during orthodontic treatment. Am J Orthod Dentofacial Orthop. 124: 206 – 211(2003)

Seymour A. R., Effects of medications on the periodontal tissues in health and disease, *Periodontol 2000.* 40: 120 – 129 (2006)

Shah P., Midha K. K., Dighe S., McGilveray J. I, Skelly P. J, Yacobi A., Layloff T.,Viswanathan C. T., Cook E. C., Mcdowall R. D., Pittman A. K., Spector S., Analytical Method Validation: Bioavailability, Bioequivalence and Pharmacokinetics Studies, J. Pharm. Sci. 8: 309-312(1992)

Shah P. V, Midha K. K., Findlay W. A. J., Hill M. H., Hulse D. J., Mcgilveray J. I.,
Mckay G., Miller J. K., Patnaik N. R., Powell L. M., Tonelli A., Viswanathan C. T., Yacobi A., Bioanalytical Method Validation–A Revisit With a Decade of Progress, Pharm. Res. 17 (12): 1551 -1557(2000)

Sheiham A., Oral health, general health and Quality of life, Bull. WHO. 83: 641-720 (2005)

Shimada K., Mitamura K., Higashi T., Gas chromatography and high performance liquid chromatography of natural steroids, J. Chrom A. 935: 141-172 (2001)

Silva F., Gomes S., Validation of an alternative absorbent paper for collecting gingival crevicular fluid, R. Periodontia 19 (3): 85-90 (2009)

Shou M., Galinada A.W., Wei Y., Tang Q., Markovic J.R., Rustum M.A., Developement and validation of a stability-indicating method for simultaneous determinationof salycilic acid,betamethasone dipropionate and their related compounds in Diprosalic Lotion®, J. Pharm. Biomed. Anal. 50: 356-361 (2009).

Scwach –Abdellaoui R., Vivien-Castioni N., Gurny R., Local delivery of antimicrobial agents for the treatment of periodontal diseases, Eur. J. Pharm. Biopharm. 50: 83-99 (2000).

Shaddox L., Walker C., Treating chronic periodontitis: current status, challenges and future directions, Clin. Cosm. Investig. Dent. 2: 79-91 (2010).

Shu P.Y., Chou S.H., Lin C.H., Determination of corticosteron in rat and mouse plasma by gas chromatography-selected ion monitoring mass spectrometry, J. Chrom. B. 783: 93-101 (2003)

Slots J., Ting M., Systemic antibiotics in the treatment of periodontal disease. Periodontol. 2000. 28: 106-176 (2002)

Souza J., Ross Junior C., garlet G., Nogueira A., Cirreli J., Modulation of the host cell signaling pathways as a therapeutic approach in periodontal disease, J. Appl. Oral Sci. 20 (2): 128-138 (2012)

Soskolne W.A., Chajek T., Flashner M., Landau I., Stabholc A., Kolatch B., Lerner E.I., An in vivo study of the chlorhexidine release profile of the PerioChip in the gingival crevicular fluid, plasma and urine, J. Clin. Periodontol. 25(12):1017-1021 (1998).

Tariq M., Iqbal Z., Ali J., Baboota S., Talegaonkar S., Ahmad Z., Sahni K. J., Treatment modalities and evaluation models for periodontitis, Int. J. Phar. Invest. 2: 106-122 (2012)

Thienpont L. M., Standardization of steroid immunoassays–in theory an easy task, Clin. Chem. Lab. Med. 36:349-352 (1998)

Tomasi C., Wennström L.J., Locally delivered doxycycline as an adjunct to mechanical debridgement at retreatment of periodontal pockets: outcome at furcation sites, J. Periodontol. 82: 210-218 (2011)

Tomson G.R., Modulating the host response as an adjunctive treatment for periodontitis, J. Periodontol. 22: 26-34 (2001)

Tözum T. F., Hatipoglu H., Yamalik N., Gursel M., Alptekin N.O, Ataoglu T., Critical steps in electronic volume quantification of gingival crevicular fluid: the potential impact of evaporation, fluid retention, local conditions and repeated measurement, J. Periodont. Res. 39: 344-357 (2004)

Tsai C.C., Kao C.C., Chen C.C., Gingival crevicular fluid lactoferrin levels in adult periodontitis, Aust Dent J. 43: 40 – 44 (1998) Vairale S., Sivaswaroop P., Bandana S., Development and validation of stability-indicating HPLC method for betamethasone dipropionate and related substances in topical formulation, Ind J Pharm. Sci. 74: 107-15 (2012)

Vienneau D.S. & Kindberg C.G., Developement and validation of a sensitive method for tetracycline in gingival crevicular fluid by HPLC using fluorescence detection, J. Pharm. Biomed. Anal. 16: 111-117 (1997).

Xiao P.K., Xiong Y., Rustum A., Quantitation of trace betamethasone and dexamethasone in dexamethasone or betamethasone active pharmaceutical ingredients by reversed-phase high performance liquid chromatography. J. Chrom Sci. 46 (1): 15-22 (2008)

Zhang J., Kashket S., Lingstrom P., Evidence for the early oneset of gingival inflammation following short-term plaque accumulation, J. Clin. Periodontol. 29: 1082-1085 (2002)

Zia A., Khan S., Gupta N. D., Muktar Un Nisar S., Oral biomarkers in the diagnosis and progression of periodontal diseases. Biol. Med. 3(2): 45-52 (2011)

Zou J.J, Dai L., Ding L., Xiao DW., Bin ZY, Fan HW, Liu L., Wang GJ., Determination of betamethasone and betamethasone-17-monopropionate in human plasma by liquid chromatography-positive/negative electrospray ionization tandem mass spectrometry, J. Chrom. B Analyt. Technol. Biomed. Life Sci. 873 (2): 159-64 (2008)

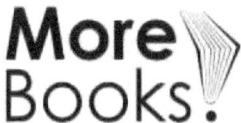

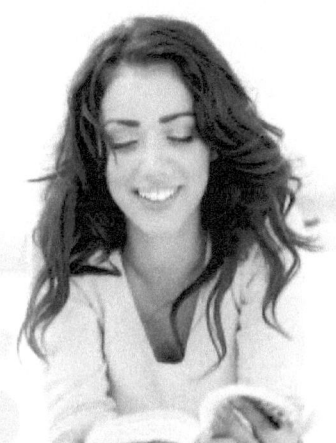

I want morebooks!

Buy your books fast and straightforward online - at one of world's fastest growing online book stores! Environmentally sound due to Print-on-Demand technologies.

Buy your books online at
www.morebooks.shop

Kaufen Sie Ihre Bücher schnell und unkompliziert online – auf einer der am schnellsten wachsenden Buchhandelsplattformen weltweit! Dank Print-On-Demand umwelt- und ressourcenschonend produziert.

Bücher schneller online kaufen
www.morebooks.shop

KS OmniScriptum Publishing
Brivibas gatve 197
LV-1039 Riga, Latvia
Telefax: +371 686 204 55

info@omniscriptum.com
www.omniscriptum.com

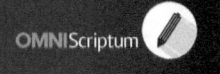

www.ingramcontent.com/pod-product-compliance
Lightning Source LLC
Chambersburg PA
CBHW020455220526
45464CB00002B/996